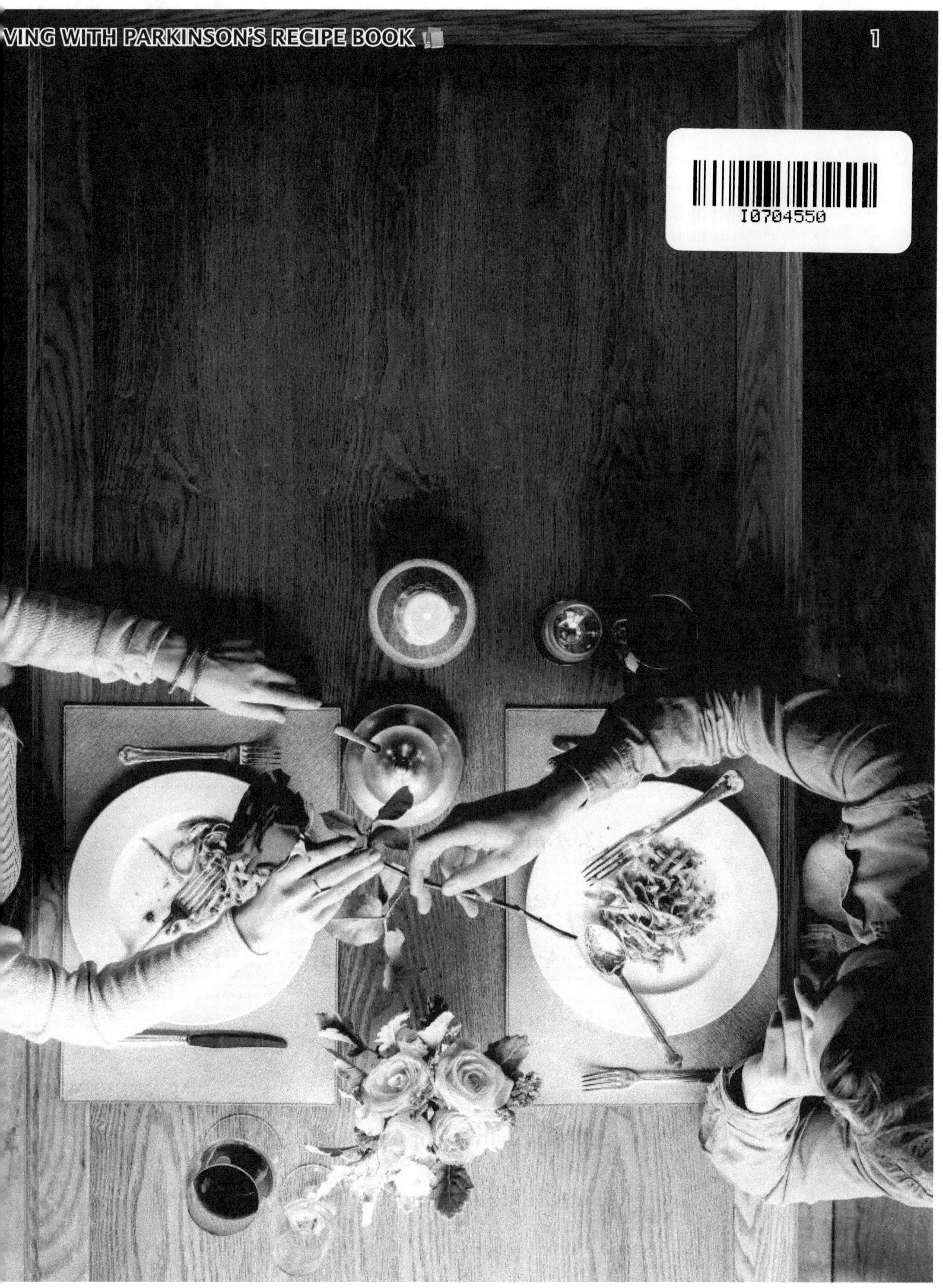

TABLE OF CONTENT

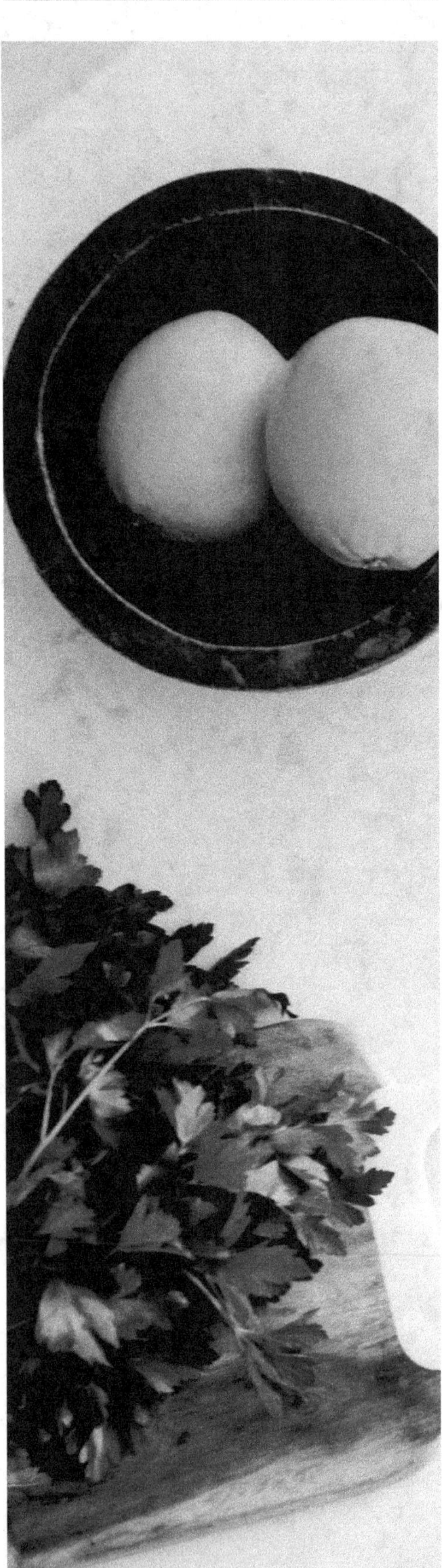

TABLE OF CONTENTS

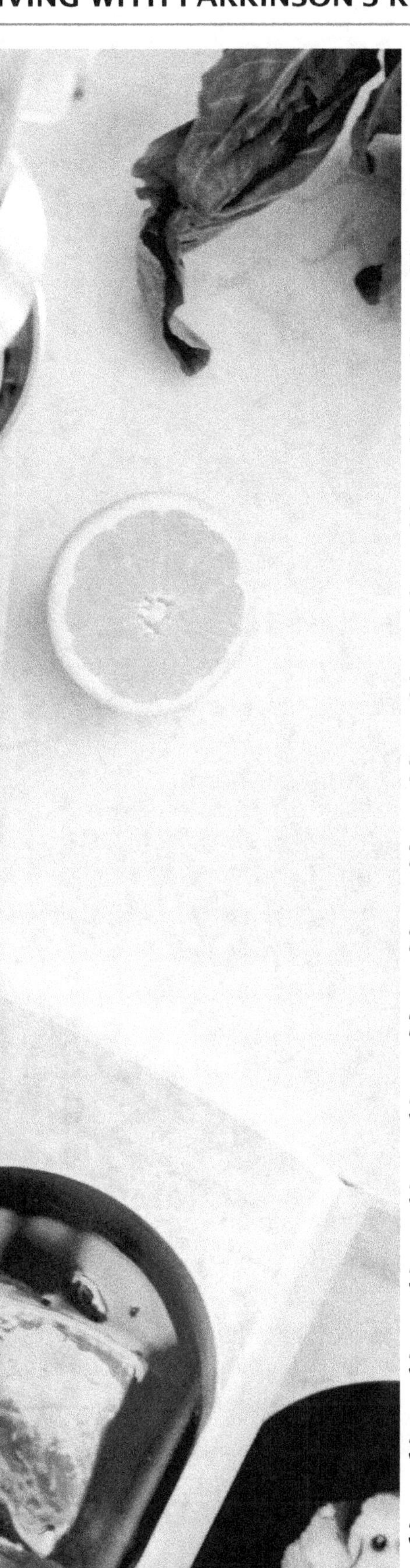

PARKINSON'S DISEASE RECIPES

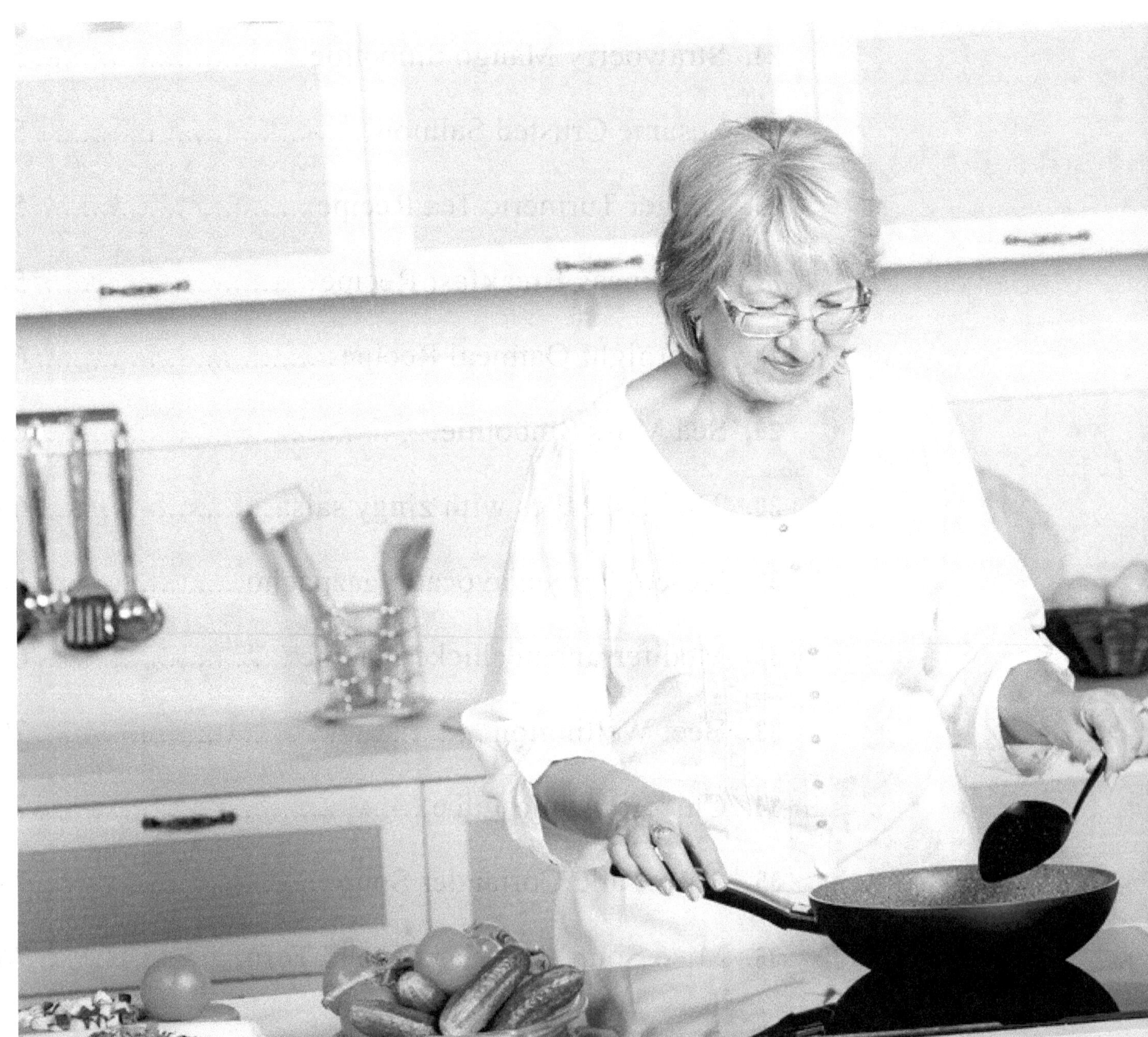

FORWARD

Parkinson's disease is a brain disorder that causes unintended or uncontrollable movements, such as shaking, stiffness, and difficulty with balance and coordination. Symptoms usually begin gradually and worsen over time. As the disease progresses, people may have difficulty walking and talking.

Following a balanced diet improves general well-being and boosts your ability to deal with symptoms of the disease. Eating plenty of whole foods, such as fruits and vegetables, lean protein, beans and legumes, and whole grains, and staying hydrated are key ways to stay energized and healthy overall.

Smoothies and juices can aslo play an important roles because it contians Vitamin C is essential for the brain development and has neuroprotective mechanisms for people with Parkinson's. Fruits rich in vitamin C include Oranges, Kiwi, Strawberries, raspberries, blueberries and cranberries.

Flourless Oatmeal Banana Nut Muffins

Ready In About 30 min

Servings 04

Ingredients

- 2 cups quick oats, or rolled oats
- 2 cups mashed ripe banana
- 2 eggs
- 2 tsp ground cinnamon
- 1 tsp baking soda
- 1/2 tsp sea salt
- 1/2 cup raw walnuts, chopped
- 1/2 cup chocolate chips, optional

Direction

01. Preheat the oven to 350 degrees F and spray oil a muffin tray.

02. Add the oats to a blender and blend until a flour forms. It's okay if it doesn't reach the consistency of regular flour. I often leave mine somewhat coarse and it turns out great.

03. Add the remaining ingredients except for the walnuts (and chocolate chips if you're adding them) and blend until smooth. Stir in the walnuts (and chocolate chips if adding).

04. Fill the muffin holes ⅔ of the way up (the muffins will rise!) and if desired, top with more walnuts, chocolate chips, and/or oats.

05. Bake on the center rack of the preheated oven for 20 to 25 minutes, or until muffins are golden-brown and feel firm when gently poked.

06. Allow muffins to cool at least 30 minutes before running a butter knife along the edge of the muffin between the muffin and the tray release the muffins.

Blueberry Almond Overnight Oats

Ready In About 12 hours

Servings 01

Ingredients

- 1/2 cup rolled oats
- 1/2 cup almond milk
- 2 Tbs. almond butter
- 1/2 tsp. vanilla extract
- 1/2 tsp. ground cinnamon
- 1 cup frozen blueberries, divided
- 1 Tbs. toasted sliced almonds

Direction

01. In mason jar combine oats, almond milk, almond butter, vanilla and cinnamon.

02. Stir in ½ cup blueberries.

03. Top with remaining ½ cup blueberries and sliced almonds.

04. Refrigerate 4 hours-overnight.

05. Stir and enjoy!

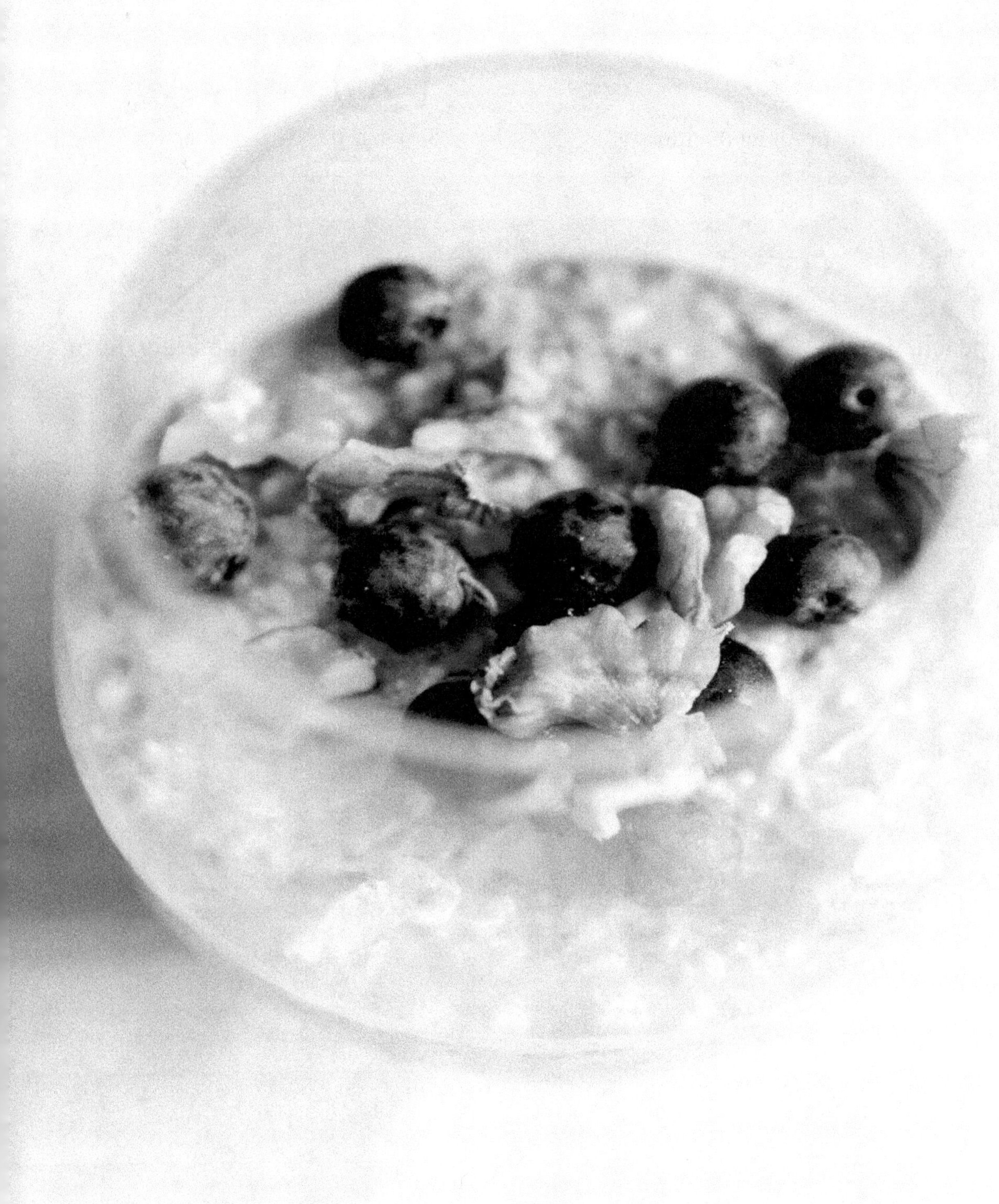

Kiwi Peach Juice

Ready In About 05 min

Servings 02

Ingredients

- 1 medium peach, pitted.
- 1 kiwi, peeled.
- 2 cups fresh spinach leaves.
- ¼ avocado.
- 150 ml cold water

Direction

01. Add all the ingredients in the electric mixer order.

02. After that, mix at high speed for 30-60 second until there is a smooth juice.

03. Enjoy!

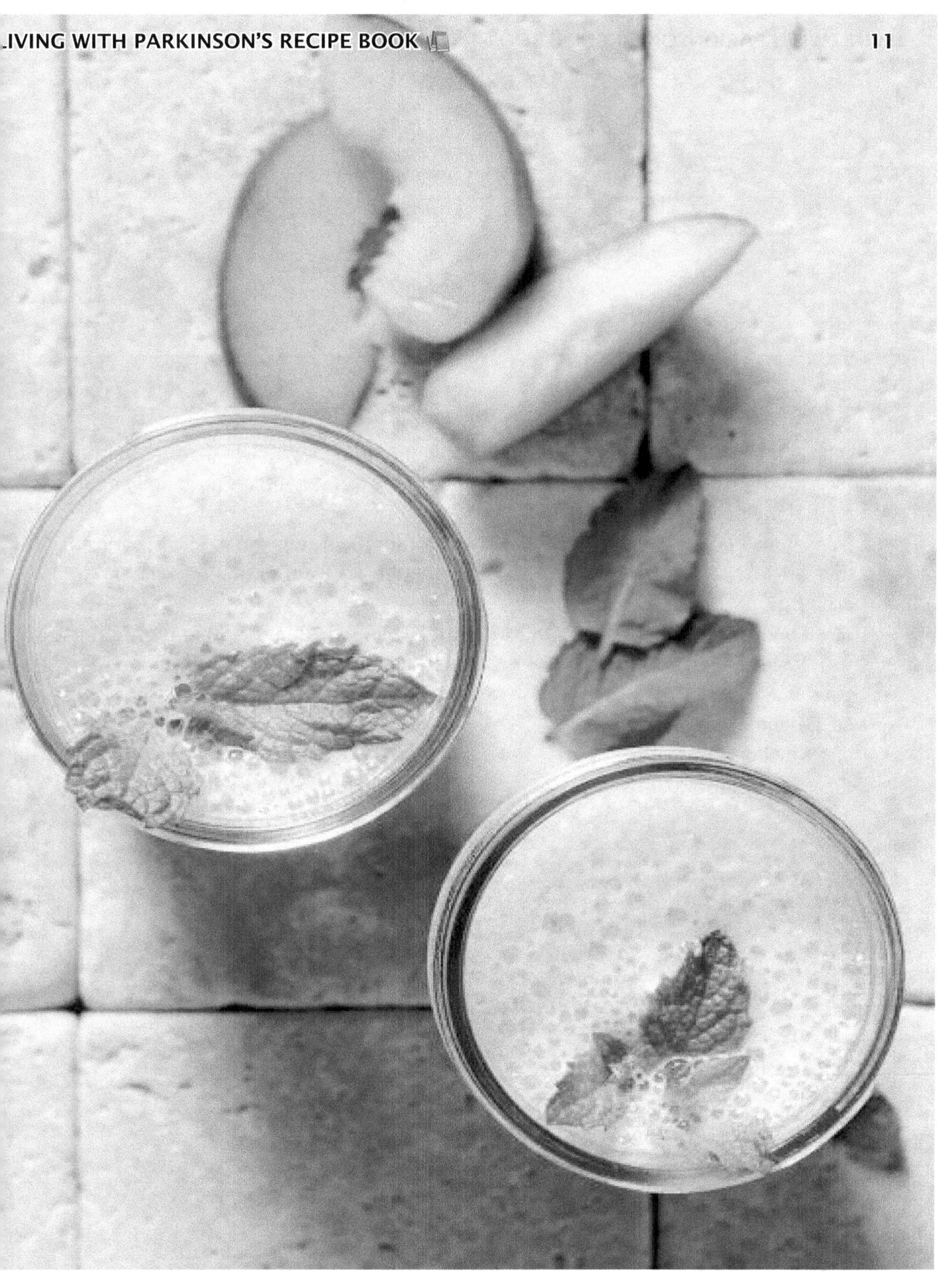

Blueberry Pancakes

Ready In About 25 min

Servings 05

Ingredients

- 1 cup Gluten free all-purpose flour
- 2 tsp Baking powder
- 1 tsp Xanthan gum
- 2 tbsp Sugar
- 1 each Egg
- 1 cup Almond milk
- 2 tbsp Vegetable oil
- 1 tsp Vanilla extract
- 1 each Lemon, zest and juice
- 1 cup Blueberries, fresh
- 2 tbsp Butter, melted

Direction

01. In a medium bowl, whisk together the flour, baking powder, xanthan gum and sugar.

02. In a small bowl, mix egg, almond milk, vegetable oil, vanilla, lemon zest and juice.

03. Add wet ingredients to dry ingredients all at once and whisk until combined. Stir in fresh blueberries.

04. Heat non-stick skillet on medium-high heat and brush pan with a little melted butter.

05. Pour ¼ cup (60 mL) of batter onto frying pan and cook until bottom is brown and bubbles appear on top.

06. Flip pancake and cook for another 1-2 minutes until cooked through.

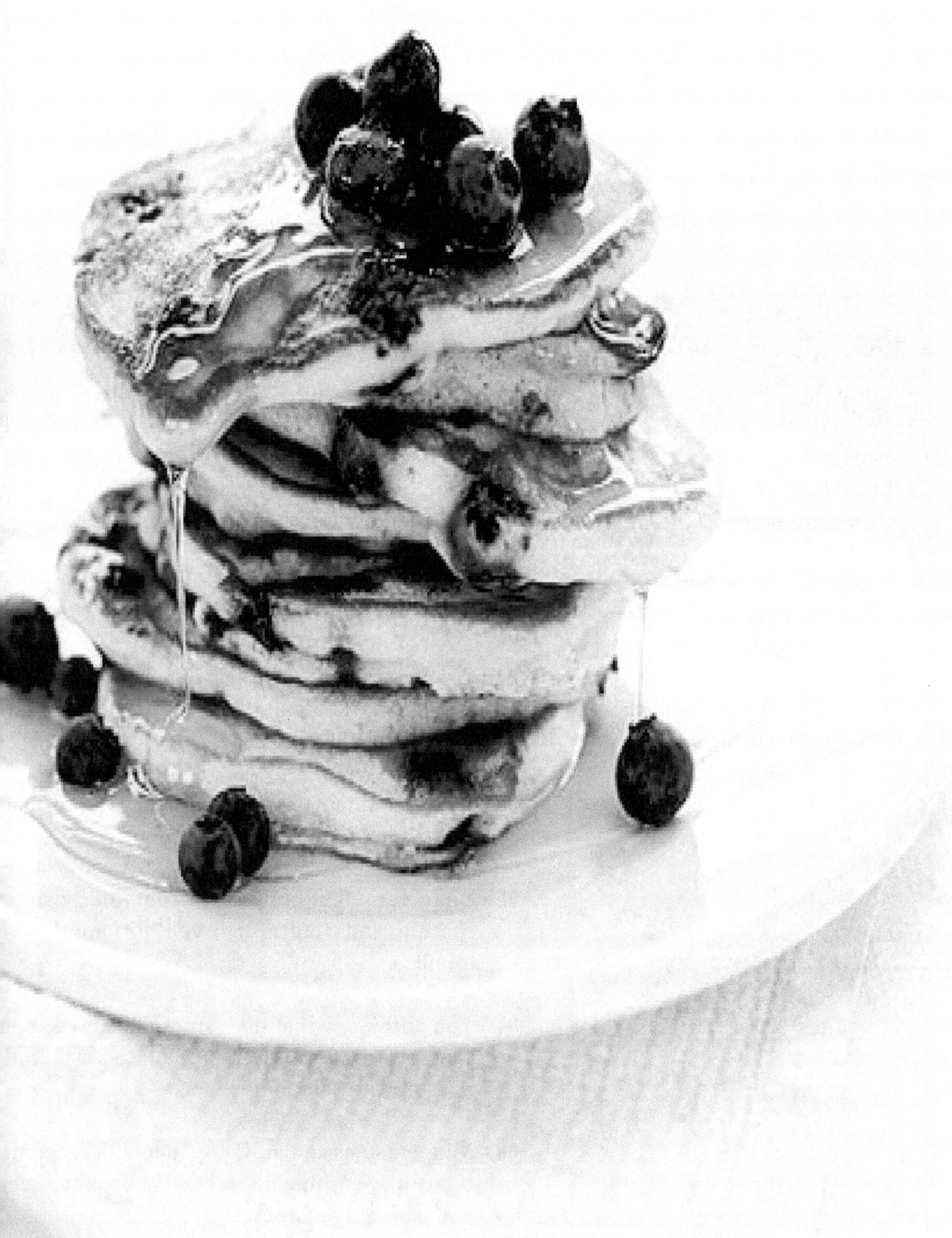

Roasted Potatoes & Tomatoes

Ready In About 25 min

Servings 06

Ingredients

- 1 tbsp Baking soda
- 3 each Russet potatoes, ½ inches diced
- 1 tbsp Paprika
- 1 tsp Salt
- 1 tbsp Olive oil
- 1 each Red pepper, thinly sliced
- 1 each Red onion, thinly sliced
- 1 pint Cherry tomatoes, cut in half
- 3 sprigs Basil leaves, chopped
- To taste Salt and pepper

Direction

01. Preheat oven to 475°F (240°C). Line a larg baking tray with parchment paper and set asid

02. Bring a large pot of water to boil. Add bakir soda and potatoes to the boiling water.

03. Allow water to return to a boil and cook for minutes.

04. Drain potatoes and transfer to a mixing bow Add paprika, salt and 1 tbsp olive oil. Mix unt potatoes are evenly coated.

05. Toss potatoes with peppers and onions ar place onto the prepared baking tray.

06. Bake for 10 minutes, flip potatoes using spatula and return to oven for another 1 minutes

07. You will know that they are finished when yc can stick a knife into the potatoes very easil Season with salt and pepper.

08. Mix tomatoes and basil together with remainir olive oil. Season with salt and pepper and serv with roasted potatoes.

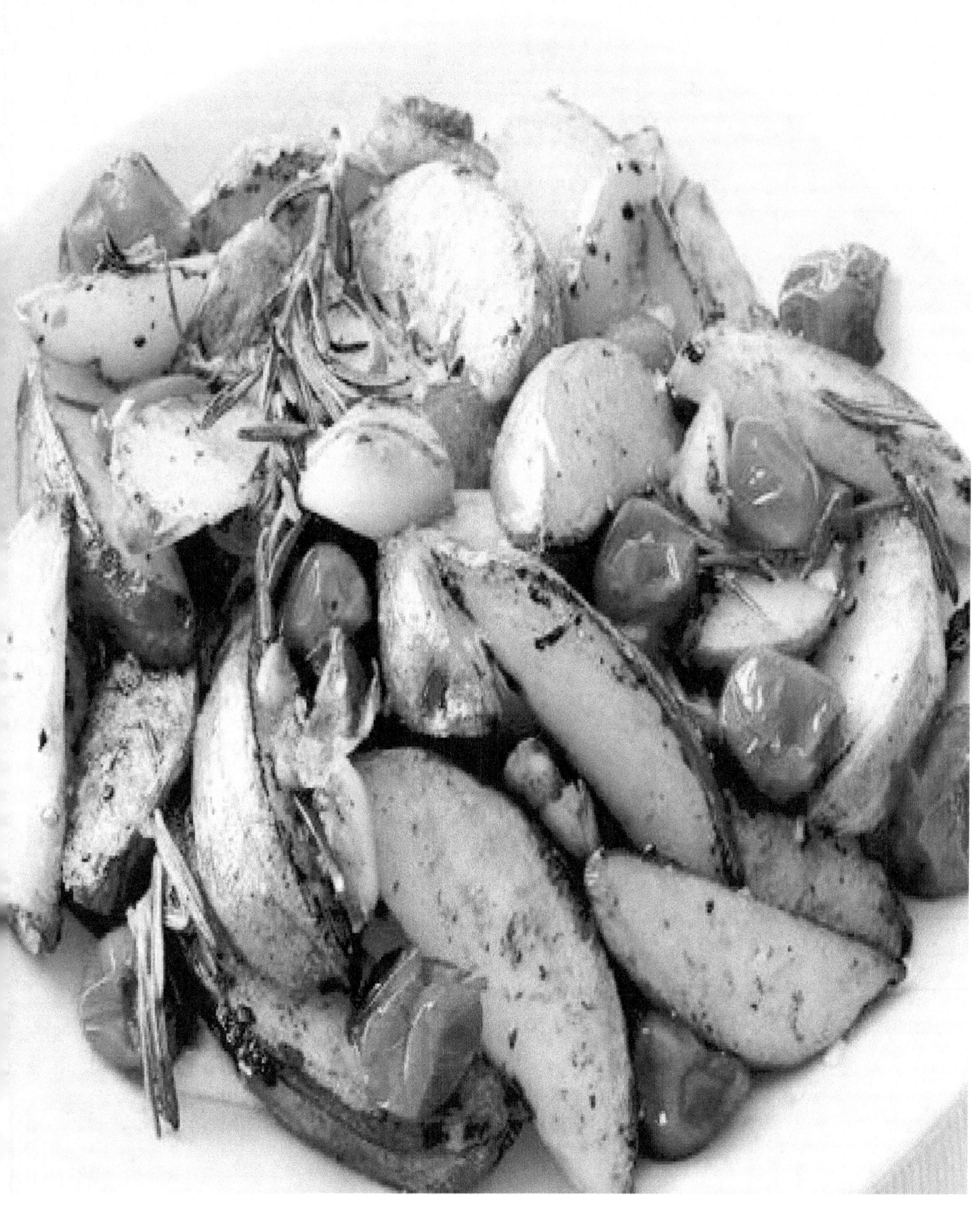

Zucchini & Chocolate Cranberry Muffins

Ready In About 25 min

Servings 12

Ingredients

- 1 ½ cup Gluten free all-purpose flour
- 2 tsp Baking powder
- ½ tsp Baking soda
- ¾ tsp Xanthan gum
- ¼ cup Brown sugar
- ¾ cup Almond milk
- 2 tbsp Honey
- 1 each Egg
- 1 tsp Vanilla extract
- 1 cup Zucchini, finely grated
- 1 cup Dried cranberries
- ½ cup Dark chocolate chips

Direction

01. Preheat oven to 375°F (190°C). Line muffin tins with paper muffin cups and set aside.

02. Melt butter in microwave and set aside to cool.

03. In a large bowl, combine flour, baking powder, baking soda, xanthan gum and sugar mix thoroughly.

04. In a separate bowl, mix the almond milk, egg, cooled butter and vanilla extract.

05. Mix wet ingredients into the dry ingredients until smooth.

06. Gently mix in the grated zucchini, cranberry, dark chocolate chips until just incorporated. Batter should be lumpy.

07. Divide the batter evenly among the muffin cups.

08. Bake for 25-30 minutes, until a toothpick inserted into the centre comes out clean, and muffins are lightly browned.

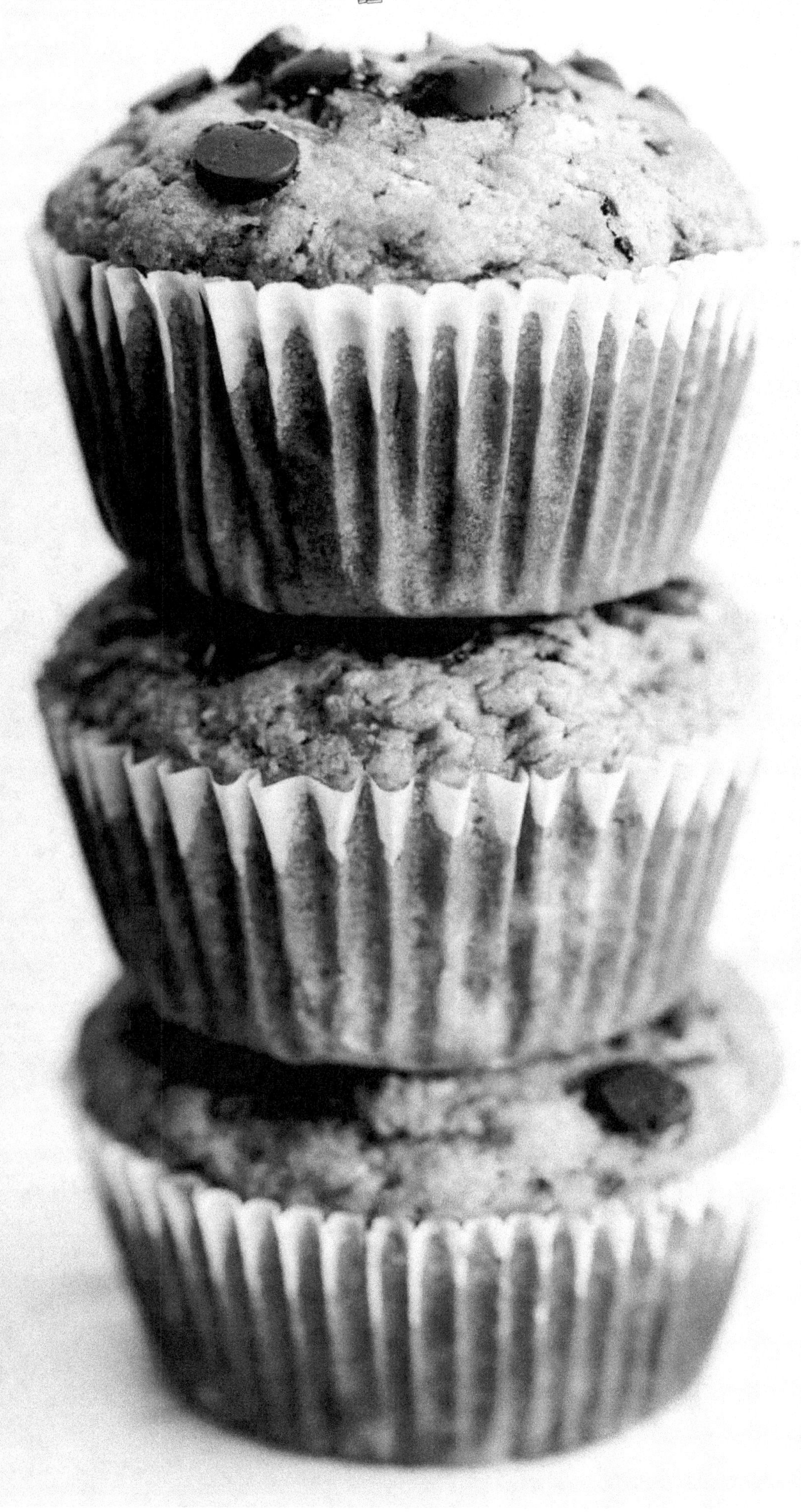

Creamy Papaya Berries Juice

Ready In About 05 min

Servings 02

Ingredients

- 1 cup papaya, diced and free from the seeds.
- 1 cup cranberry.
- 2 cups fresh spinach or any green leaves as desired.
- 150 ml cold water.

Direction

01. Add all the ingredients in the electric mixer in order.

02. After that, mix at high speed for 30-60 seconds until there is a smooth juice.

03. Enjoy!

Ginger & Veg Stir-Fry

Ready In About 45 min

Servings 06

Ingredients

- 125 g Rice noodles, wide
- 1 tbsp Corn starch
- ¼ cup Vegetable oil
- 2 cups Broccoli florets, bite-sized
- 1 each Carrot, thinly sliced half-moon shape
- 1 pkg Mushrooms, quartered
- 1 each Red pepper, thinly sliced
- 1 each Yellow pepper, thinly sliced
- ½ cup Snow peas, stem removed
- 1 each Onion, sliced
- 1 clove Garlic, grated
- 2 tsp Ginger, grated
- 3 tbsp Soy sauce, light
- 3 tbsp Water
- ½ tsp Salt

Direction

01. Bring a large pot of water to a boil and remove from heat. Put rice noodles into pot and soak until they are al dente (approximately 20-25 minutes). Check noodles periodically to make sure they do not become too soft.

02. When noodles are al dente, rinse with cold water and drain. Set aside. In a large bowl, mix cornstarch and 2 tbsp of vegetable oil together until cornstarch is dissolved.

03. Toss broccoli, carrots, mushrooms, red pepper, yellow pepper and snow peas in corn starch mixture to coat.

04. Heat the remaining oil, 2 tbsp in a large wok over medium high heat. Sauté onions, garlic and ginger with oil.

05. Add vegetables and cook for 2 minutes, stirring constantly to prevent burning. Mix soy sauce, water and salt together and add to the wok.

06. Add soaked rice noodles and gently stir fry until vegetables are cooked and tender. Do not over mix.

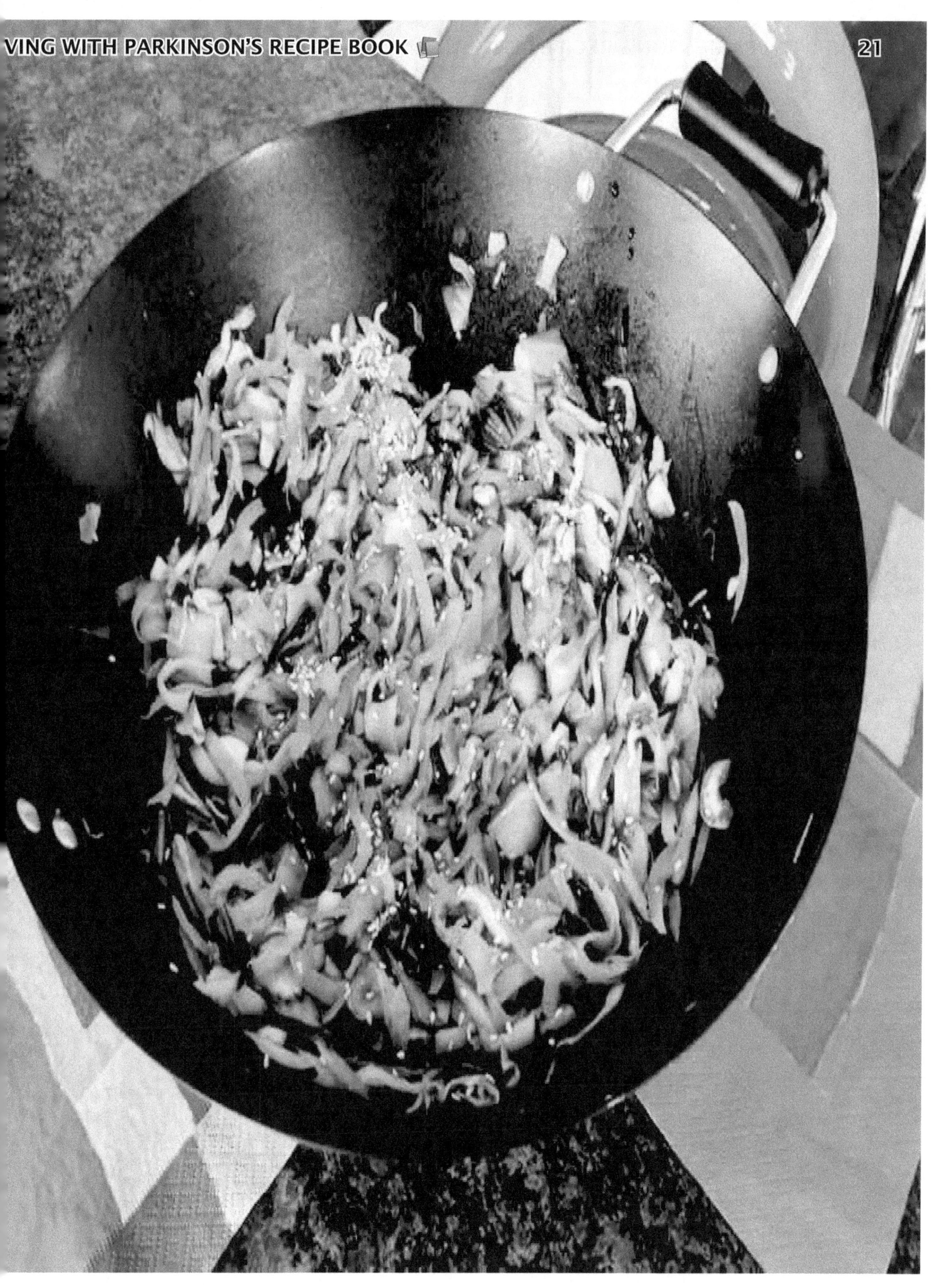

Onion Gravy

Ready In About 35 min

Servings 12

Ingredients

- 1 tbsp Butter
- 1 tbsp Vegetable oil
- 2 each Onions, finely chopped
- 1 tsp Sugar
- 1 tsp Red wine vinegar
- 2 cups Vegetable stock
- 1 tbsp Dijon mustard
- 1 pinch Black pepper
- To taste Salt

Direction

01. n a small sauce pot on low heat, melt butter an add the vegetable oil.

02. Add onions and cook on low heat until they a browned and soft. Approximately 20 minutes

03. Add sugar and cook for 2 minutes. Stir i vinegar and stock and cook for an additional 1 minutes or until gravy has reduced by half.

04. Stir in mustard and pepper. Season to taste wi salt.

05. Remove from heat and using a hand blende blend until smooth.

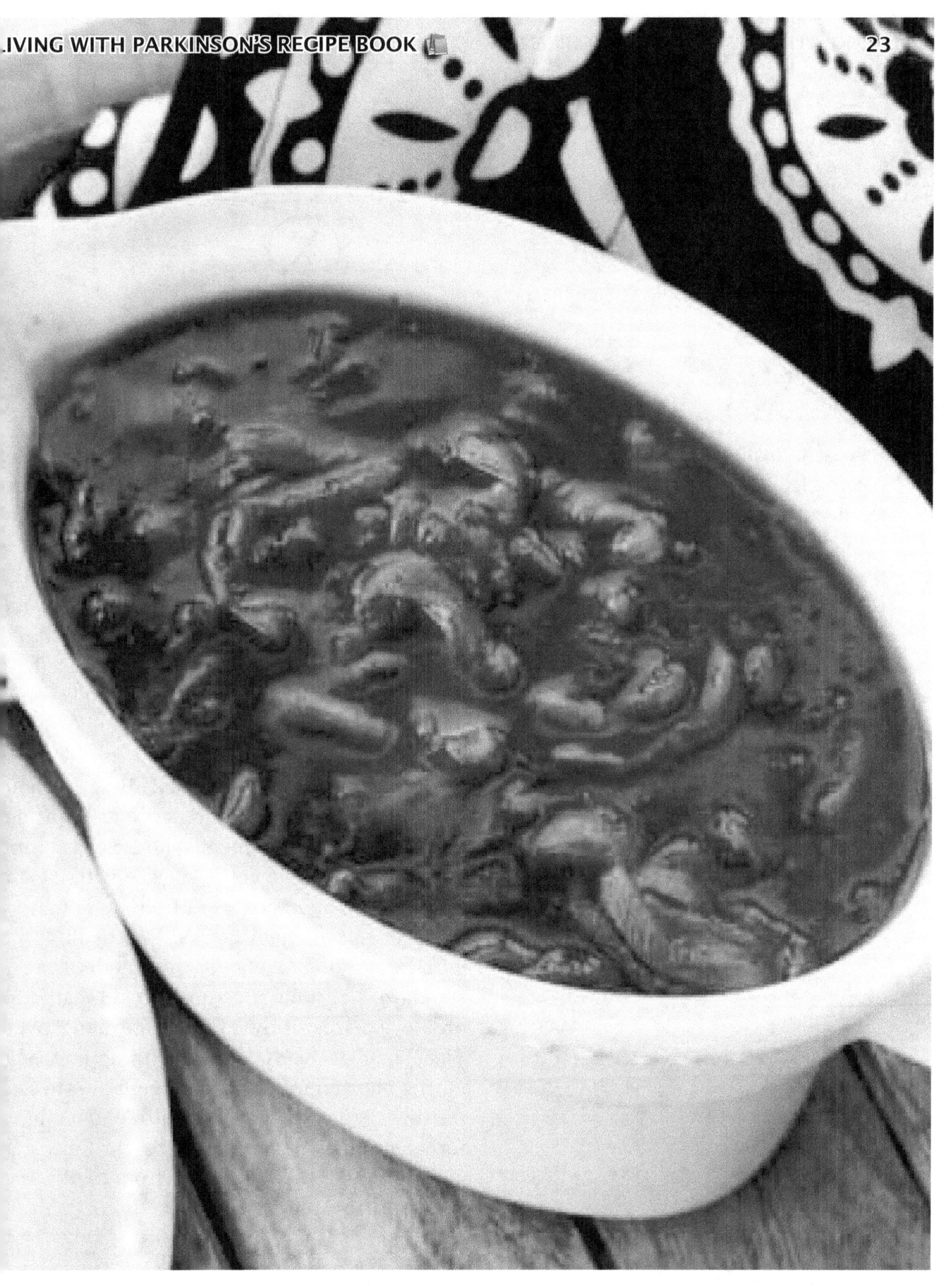

Potato & Mushroom Pie

Ready In About 10 min

Servings 03

Ingredients

- ½ each Potato, peeled and parboiled, ½ in. diced
- 2 tbsp Vegetable oil
- 1 each Onion, ½ inches diced
- 1 clove Garlic, minced
- ½ tsp Rosemary, dried
- 1 tsp Thyme, dried
- 1 cup Mushrooms, ½ in. diced
- ½ each Sweet potato, peeled and coarsely grated
- 1 tbsp Lemon juice
- To taste Salt and pepper
- 3 tbsp Butter
- 4 sheets Phyllo pastry

Direction

01. Preheat oven to 375°F. In a medium pot, bring 2 cups of water to a boil and add diced potatoes. Return to a boil and cook for 2 minutes. Drain potatoes, run under cold water and set aside. Heat oil in large skillet and add onions, garlic, rosemary and thyme. Cook until onions become translucent and add potatoes. When potatoes are golden, stir in the grated sweet potato, 1 tbsp of butter and mushrooms. Cook until mushrooms are tender and add lemon juice.

02. Season with salt and pepper and allow filling to cool. Melt the remaining butter and set aside. Lay 1 sheet of phyllo dough onto a clean cutting board and brush the entire surface with melted butter. Place another sheet of phyllo dough on top. Cut into 6 equal pieces. Repeat this step with remaining 2 sheets of dough. Line a standard size non-stick muffin tin with the phyllo squares allowing sides to hang over. Place approximately ⅓ cup of filling into each muffin cup and fold hanging dough over to seal the pies. Brush with remaining butter and bake for 15 minutes or until the pies are flaky and golden brown. Gently remove from muffin tins and allow to cool on wire rack.

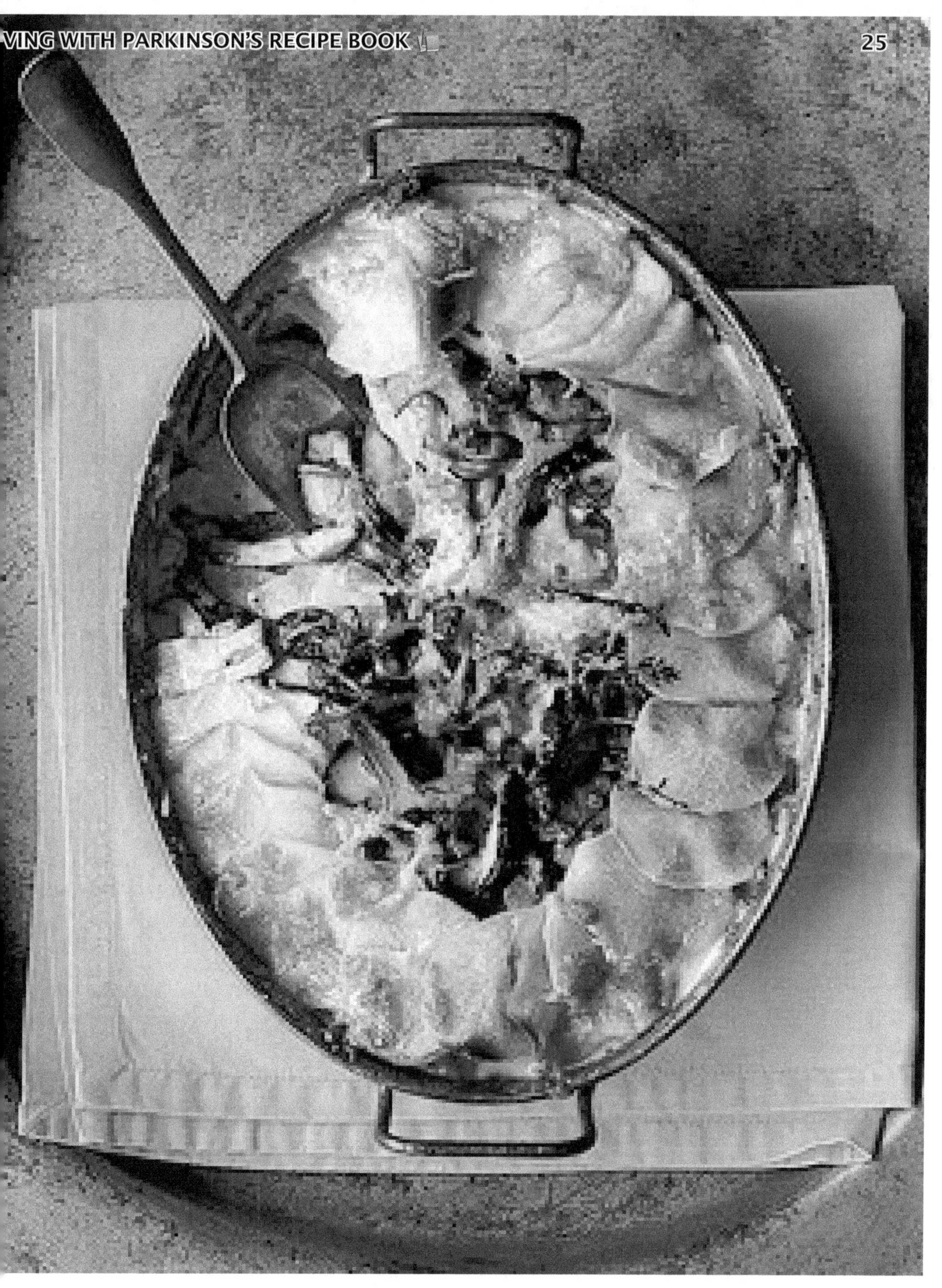

Cranberry Nectarine Juice

Ready In Abou 05 min

Servings 02

Ingredients

- 1 cup cranberry
- 1 nectarine, pitted
- 3 large strawberries
- 2 cups fresh spinach leaves
- 150 ml cold water

Direction

01. Add all the ingredients in the electric mixer i[n] order.

02. After that, mix at high speed for 30-60 second[s] until there is a smooth juice.

03. Enjoy!

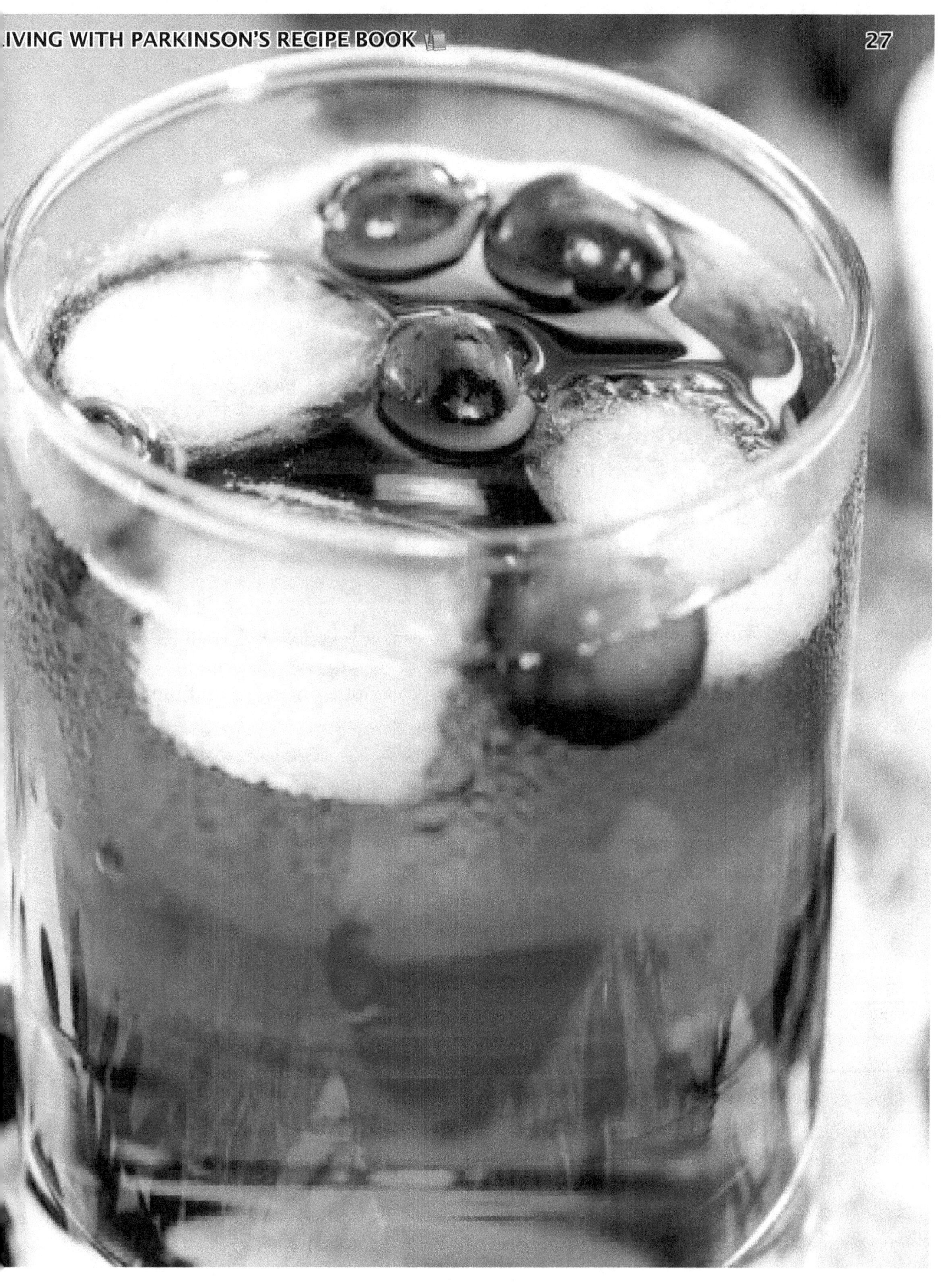

Spicy Ketchup

Ready In About 35 min

Servings 12

Ingredients

- 2 tbsp Vegetable oil
- 1 each Onion, diced
- 4 cloves Garlic, minced
- 1 each Red bell pepper, diced
- ½ cup Tomato paste
- 1 tsp Chili flakes, dried
- 2 tbsp Red wine vinegar
- ¼ cup Brown sugar, packed
- 2 tsp Salt
- 1 tsp Black pepper

Direction

01. Heat oil in a small pot. Cook onions, garlic and red bell pepper until onions are caramelized or a low heat for 10 minutes, stirring often to prevent burning.

02. Stir in tomato paste, chili flakes, vinegar and sugar. Cook for an additional 10 minutes.

03. Remove pot from stove and purée using a hand blender.

04. Season with salt and pepper

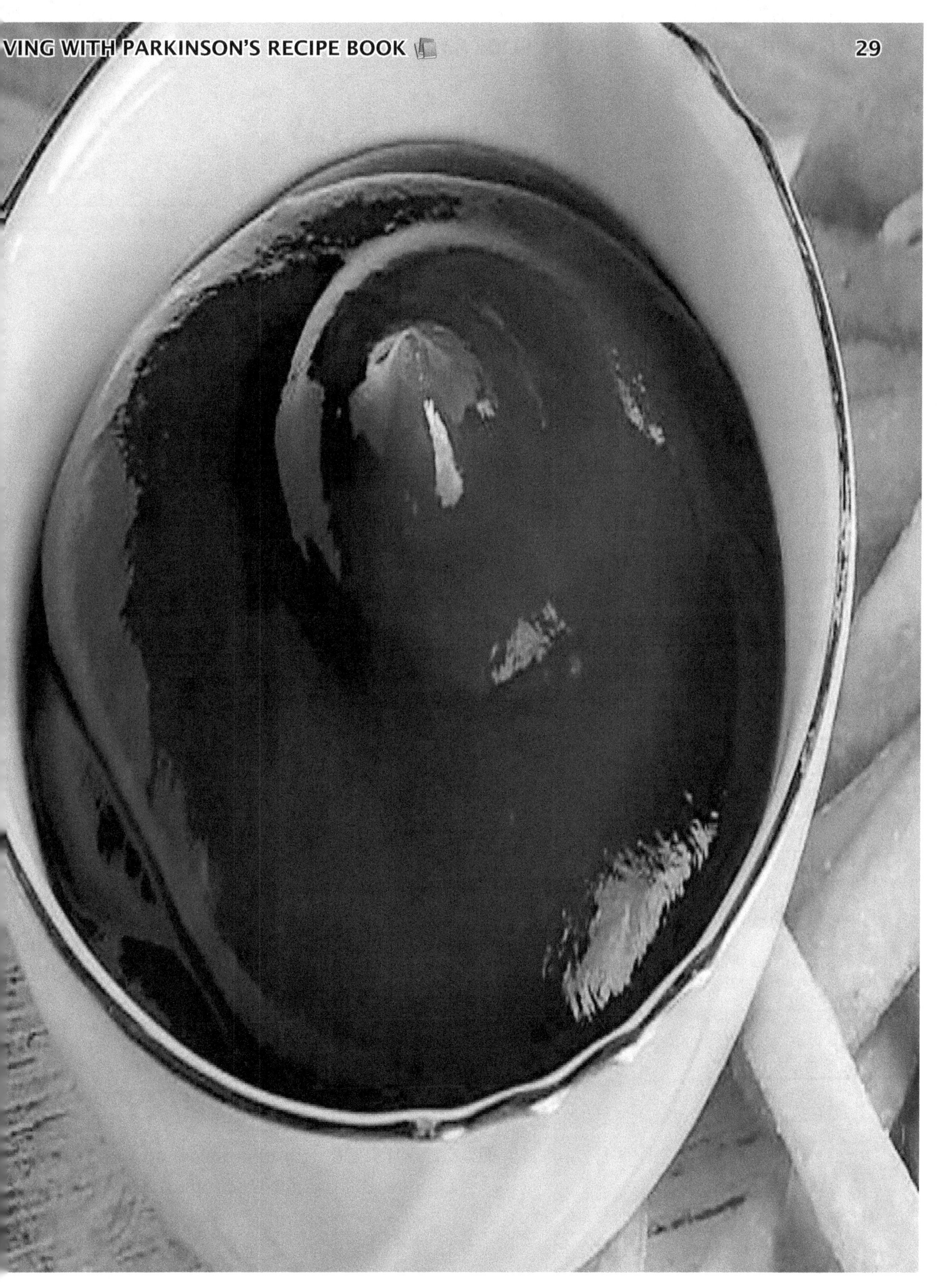

Veg Medley Stew

Ready In About 60 min

Servings 08

Ingredients

- ¼ cup Butter
- 1 each Onion, diced
- 3 each Garlic, minced
- 1 tsp Thyme, dried
- 1 tbsp Tomato paste
- ½ each Cauliflower, roughly chopped
- 3 cups Vegetable broth, low sodium
- 2 each Carrot, diced
- 1 each Red bell pepper, diced
- 2 each Zucchini, diced
- 1 can Diced canned tomatoes, with juices
- 1 tsp Salt
- ¼ tsp Black pepper

Direction

01. In a large stockpot, heat 2 tbsp of butter. Ad onions, garlic, tomato paste and thyme. Coo over a low heat, stirring occasionally, unt onions are transparent.

02. Add in cauliflower and 2 cups of stock. Brir to a boil and cook for approximately 5 minute until cauliflower is soft. Purée with han blender until smooth.

03. Heat remaining 2 tbsp of butter in a large sau pan and add carrots.

04. Cook for 2 minutes and add red bell peppe Cook until carrots and peppers are caramelize

05. Stir carrots and peppers into cauliflower pure along with zucchini and diced tomatoes. Brir to a boil.

06. Add remaining stock and salt and peppe Return to a boil and reduce to a simmer.

07. Cook for 20 minutes uncovered on a mediu heat until stew has thickened. Season to taste

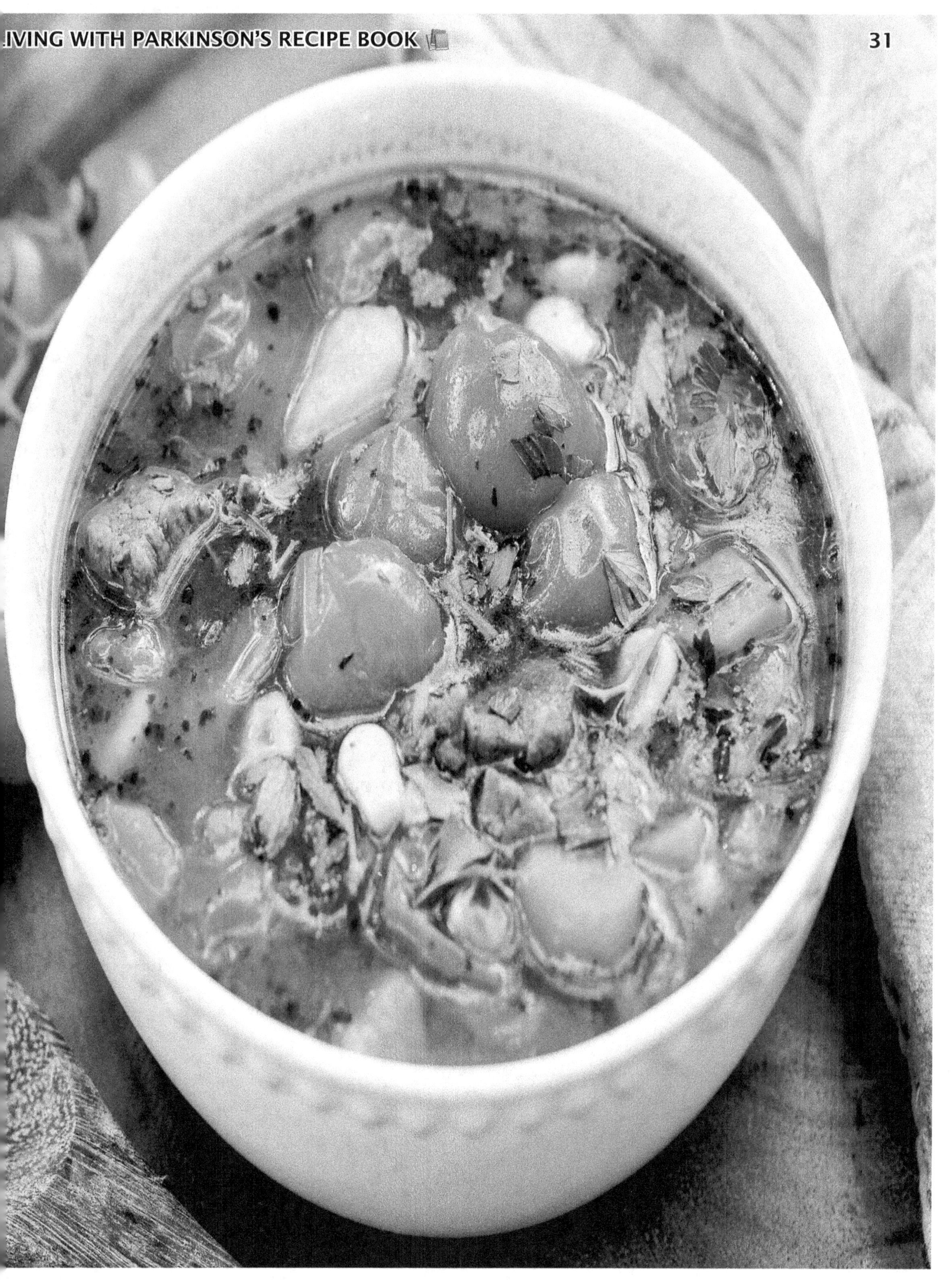

Apple Crumble Square

Ready In About 10 min

Servings 02

Ingredients

- 1½ cups All-purpose flour
- 1 tsp Baking powder
- 1 tsp Cinnamon
- ½ tsp Salt
- ½ cup Sugar
- ½ cup Brown sugar, loosely packed
- 2 each Eggs
- ⅓ cup Vegetable oil
- 1 tsp Vanilla extract
- 4 cups McIntosh apples, unpeeled, cored and ½ in. diced

Direction

01. Preheat oven to 350°F (180°C). Line a 9 x 13 in (3.5 L) pan with parchment paper and set aside

02. Sift flour, baking powder, cinnamon, and sal together in a medium bowl and set aside.

03. In a large bowl, whisk together sugar, browr sugar, eggs, vegetable oil and vanilla extrac until smooth.

04. Mix dry ingredients into wet ingredients unti just incorporated.

05. Fold apples into the batter and spread evenly with spatula onto lined baking pan.

06. To prepare topping, place the ingredients in a medium bowl and gently rub together with fingertips until crumbly.

07. Top batter with crumb topping, and bake fo 45-55 minutes.

08. Cake is ready when an inserted toothpick come out clean.

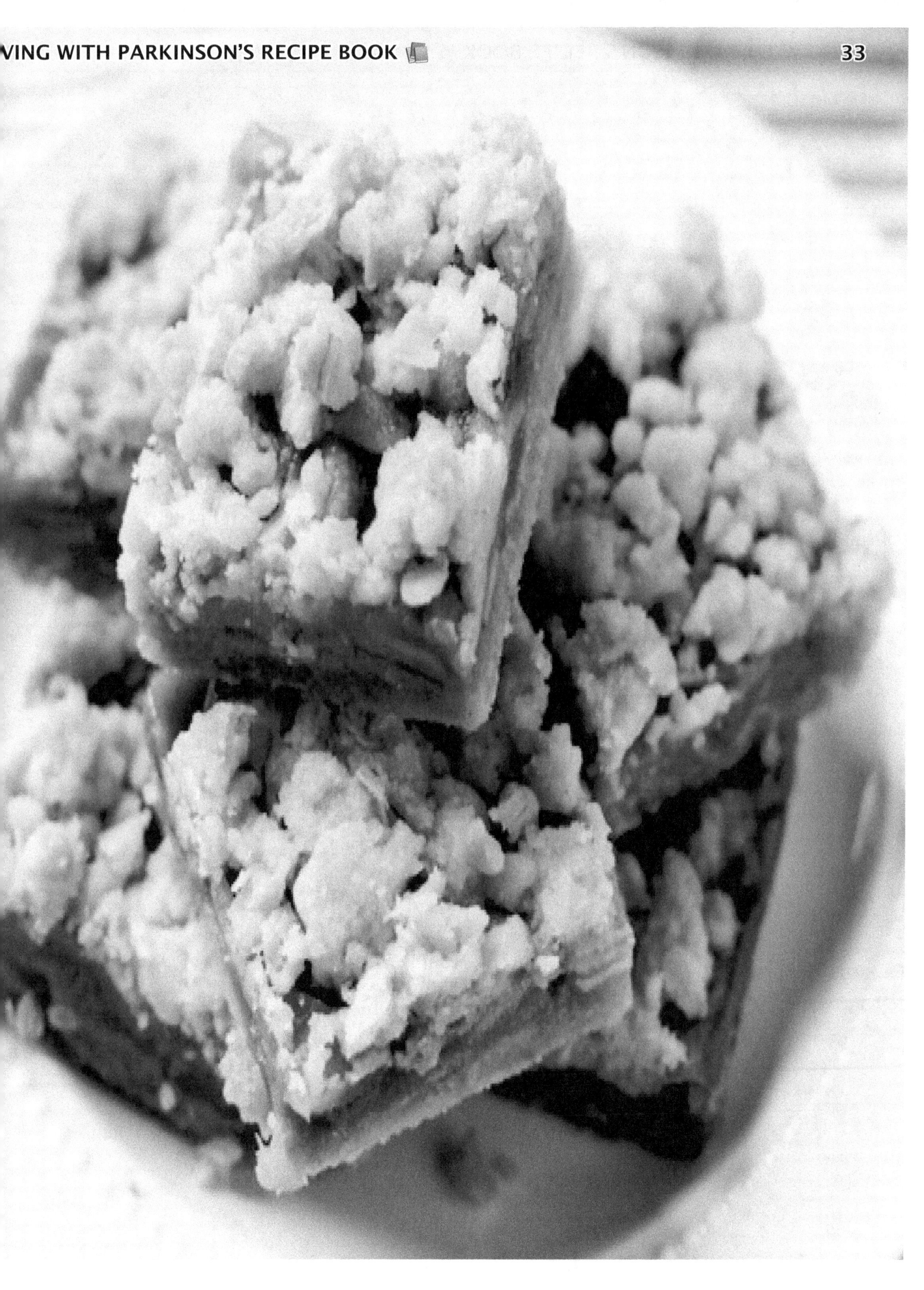

Tartar Sauce

Ready In About 5 min

Servings 03

Ingredients

- ¾ cup Mayonnaise
- ¼ cup Relish
- 1 tbsp Lemon juice
- 2 tbsp Green onion, chopped
- ¼ tsp Cayenne pepper (optional)
- 1 tsp Onion powder
- 1 each Lemon, zest and juice
- 1 each Egg
- 1 can Black beans, drained and rinsed
- 3 -213g cans Salmon, drained
- ½ cup All-purpose flour
- ¼ cup Vegetable oil

Direction

01. Combine all ingredients and mix well.

02. Refrigerate in an airtight container until read to serve

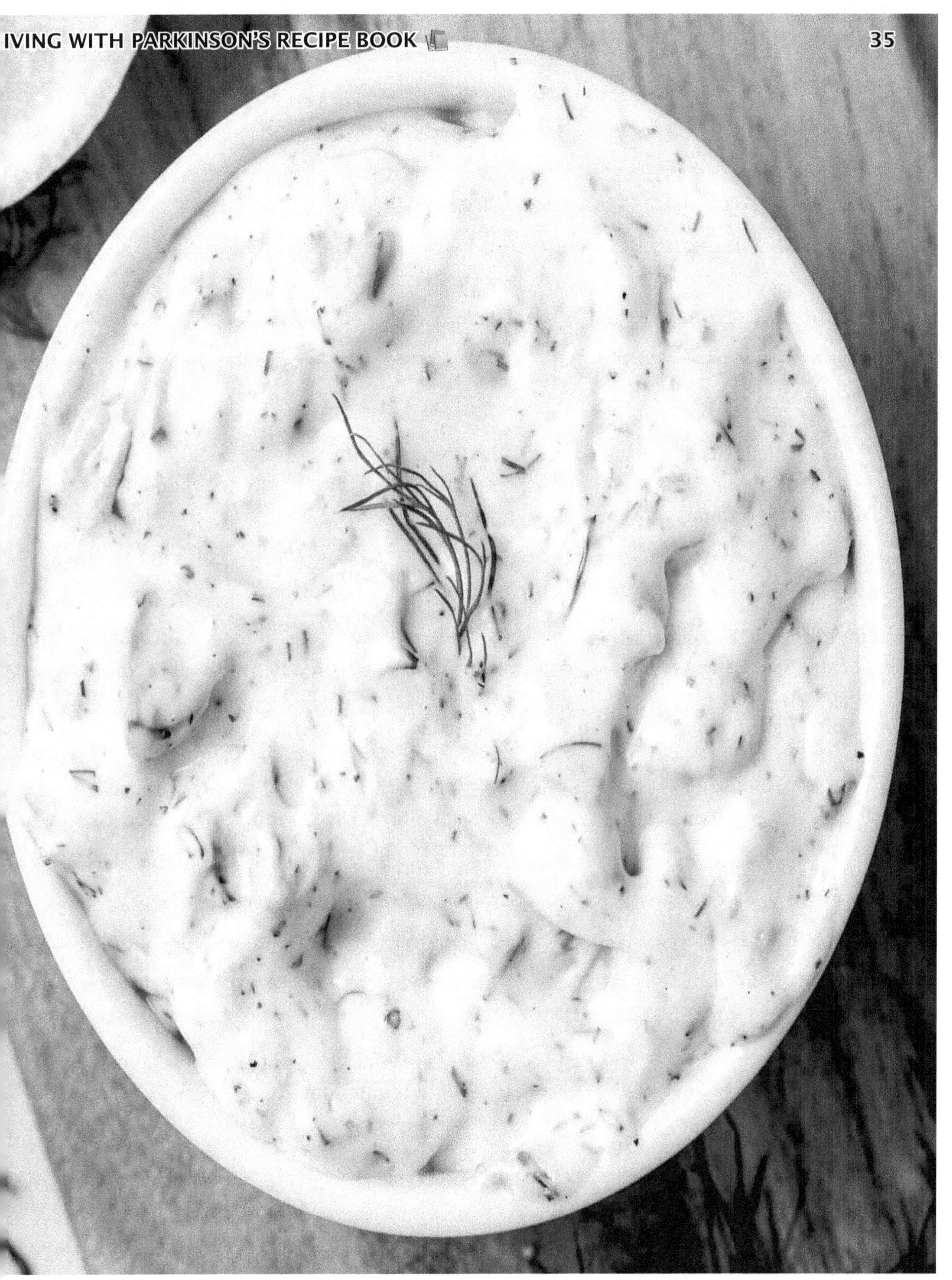

Fruit Bars

Ready In About 30 min

Servings 06

Ingredients

- ¾ cup Rolled oats, large flakes
- ½ cup All-purpose flour
- ½ cup Tapioca flour
- ½ cup Brown sugar, loosely packed
- ½ cup Dried shredded coconut, unsweetened
- ½ cup Dried apricots, finely chopped
- ½ cup Dried cranberries, roughly chopped
- ½ cup Raisins
- ½ cup Butter, softened
  Topping:
- ½ cup Semi-sweet chocolate

Direction

01. Preheat oven to 350°F (180°C). Line an 8 in square pan with parchment paper and set aside.

02. In a medium bowl, blend all the dry ingredients together with fingers.

03. Add mixture to softened butter and continue mixing with fingers until crumbly.

04. Spread into the lined baking pan and pat down firmly.

05. Bake for 15 to 20 minutes. You will know bars are ready when they are golden brown on the top.

06. Remove from oven and let cool to room temperature for 15 minutes. Refrigerate for 15 minutes until it is cold.

07. Melt chocolate in microwave and let cool to room temperature.

08. Spread onto cold fruit bars with a rubber spatula and return to refrigerator until chocolate is set. Cut into bars.

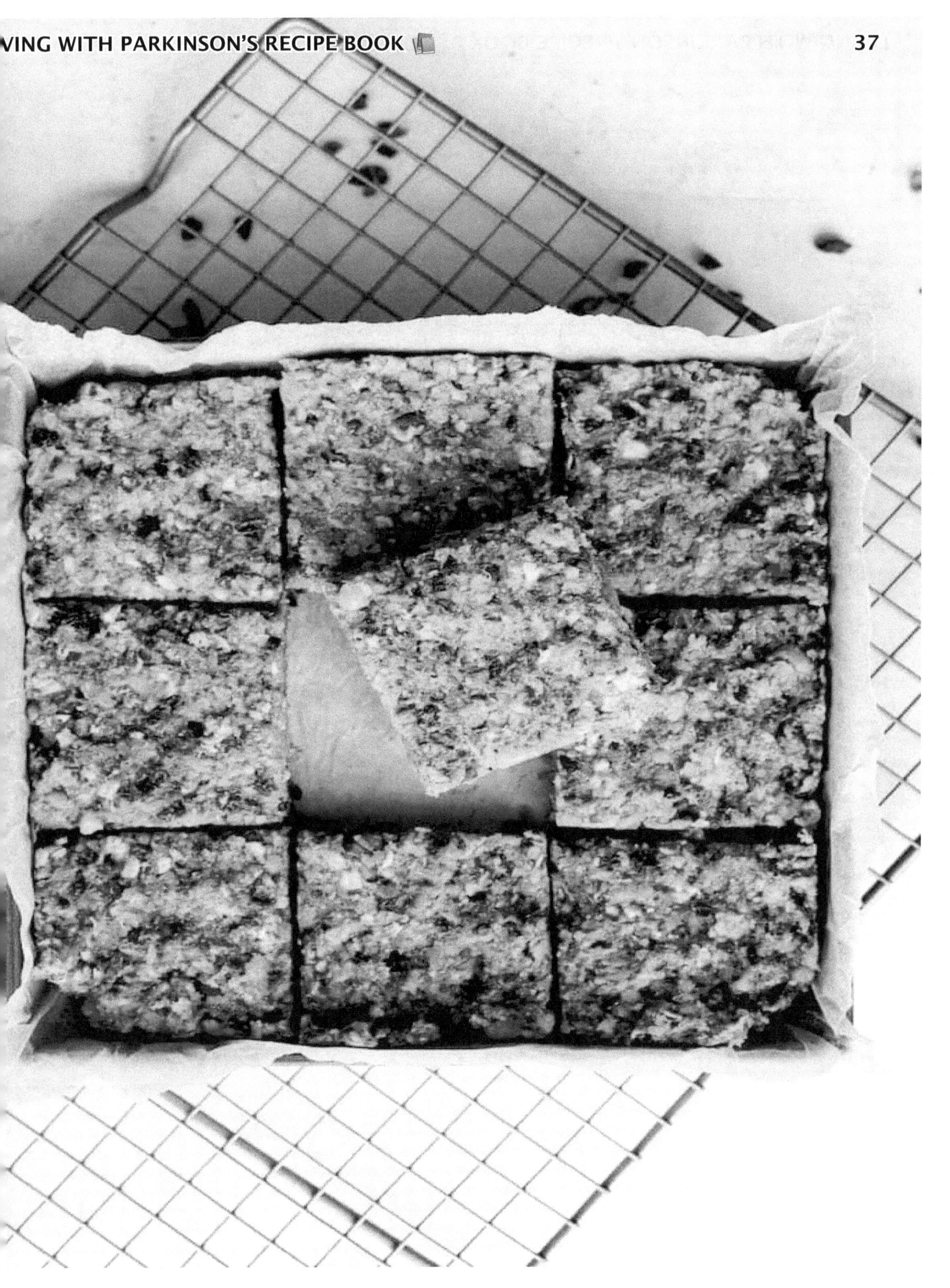

Avocado Apple Juice

Ready In About 05 min

Servings 02

Ingredients

- ¼ avocado
- 1 medium apple, with no seeds
- 2 cups chard or spinach
- 150 ml cold water.

Direction

01. Add all the ingredients in the electric mixer order.

02. After that, mix at high speed for 30-60 second until there is a smooth juice.

03. Enjoy!

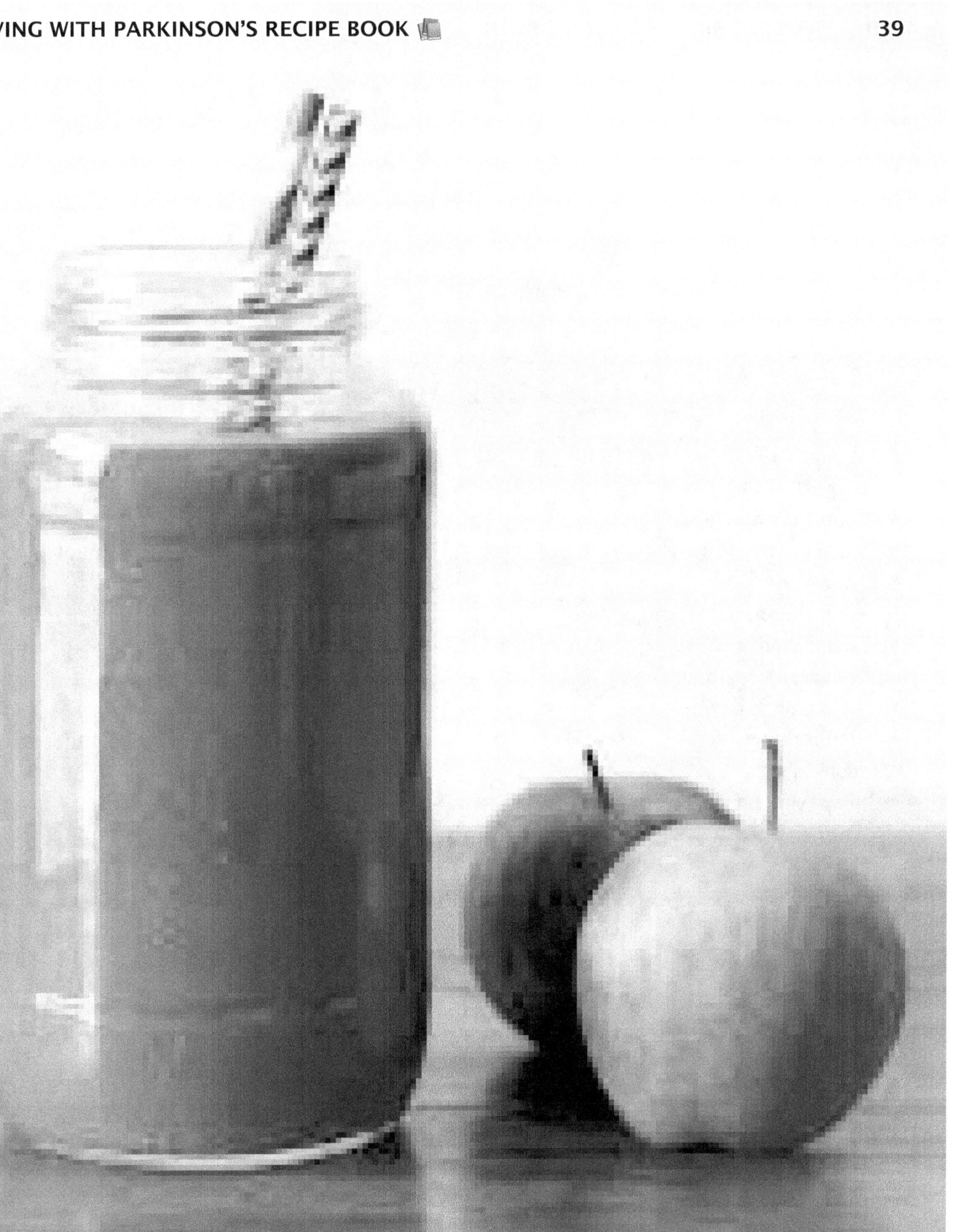

Chocolate and Orange Date Square

Ready In About 60 min

Servings 09

Ingredients

- 1¾ cup Dried dates, pitted and chopped
- ⅓ cup Maple syrup
- 1 each Orange zest
- ¾ cup Water
- ½ cup Butter, room temperature
- ½ cup Sugar
- 1½ cup Tapioca flour
- ½ cup Cocoa powder
- ¼ tsp Baking soda
- Pinch Salt
- 3 tbsp Almond milk

Direction

01. Preheat oven to 350°F (180°C). Line 8 inche square pan with parchment paper and set aside

02. In a sauce pan combine the dates, maple syrup orange zest and water.

03. Simmer until mixture thickens to a jan consistency, approximately 15 minutes.

04. In a large mixing bowl, cream together butte and sugar and set aside.

05. In a separate bowl combine the tapioca flour cocoa powder, baking soda and salt. Stir t combine.

06. Mix dry ingredients into the butter and sugar Stir in the thickened cooked dates and almon milk.

07. Spread mixture into lined pan and bake for 3(to 35 minutes. Let cool completely before slicing.

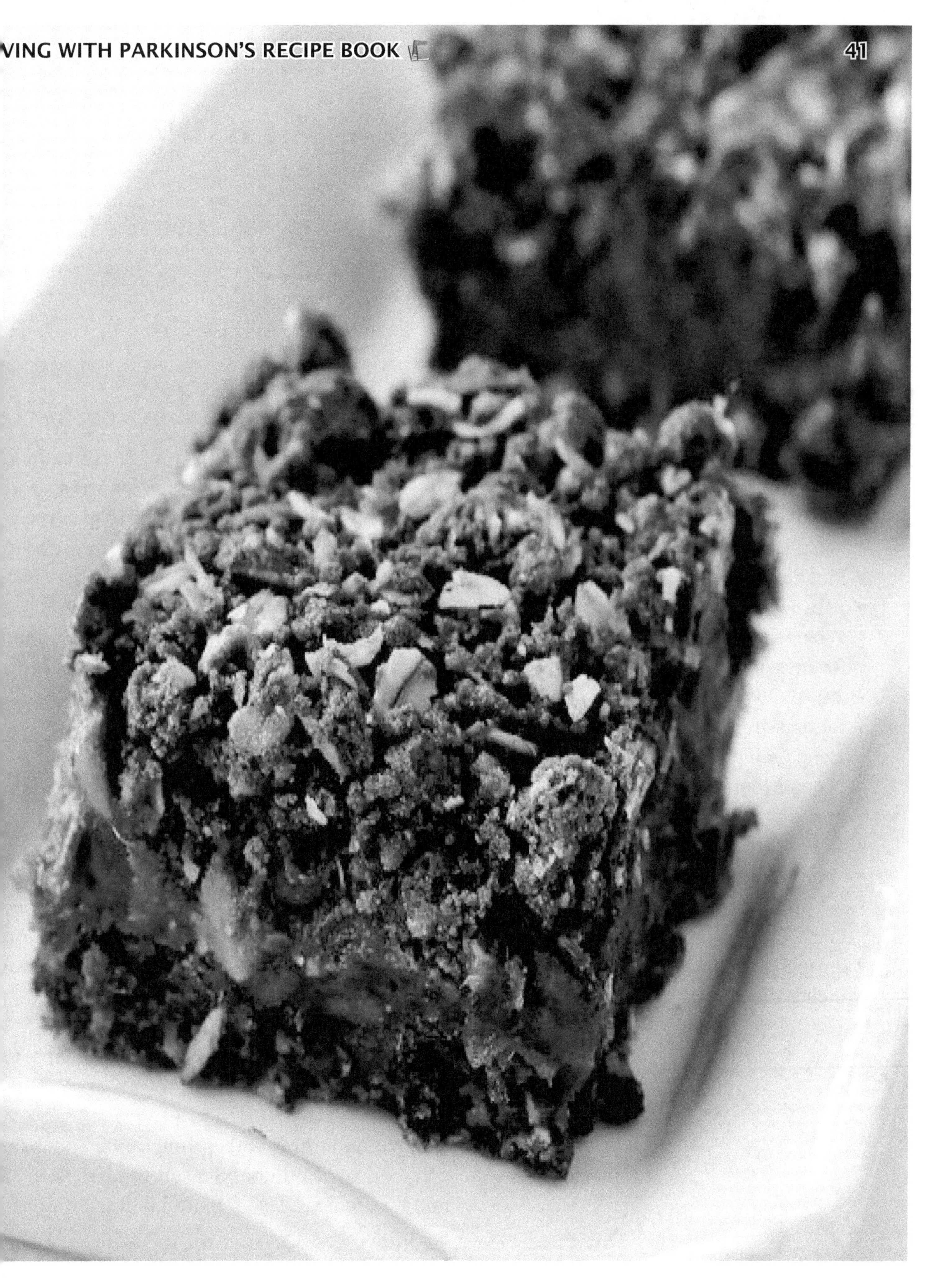

Southwestern-style Chicken & Quinoa

Ready In About 60 min

Servings 04

Ingredients

- 4 each Chicken breasts, boneless and skinless
- ¾ tsp Salt
- ¼ tsp Black pepper
- Pinch Paprika
- 1 tbsp Garlic powder
- ⅓ cup Lime juice, reserve 2 tbsp for dressing
- 2 tbsp Olive oil, reserve 1 tbsp for dressing
- 1 cup Quinoa
- ½ cup Monterey Jack cheese, grated
- 4 each Green onion, chopped
- ¾ cup Corn, canned and drained
- ¾ cup Black beans, canned and drained
- 2 each Plum tomatoes, seeded, ½ inches diced

Direction

01. Preheat oven to 350°F (180°C). Season chicke breast with salt, black pepper, paprika, garl powder, 3 tbsp lime juice and 1 tbsp olive o Transfer to baking dish and place in preheate oven.

02. Rinse quinoa under running water for 3 minut using a fine mesh sieve. Cook quinoa accordir to package instructions. Once quinoa is cooke let rest, uncovered.

03. After 15 minutes of cooking, turn over chicke and continue to cook for an additional 1 minutes.

04. After 10 minutes, sprinkle chicken breasts wi grated cheese and return to oven for an addition 3 minutes, or until cheese is melted. Remov from oven and cut into ½ in. slices.

05. Add ½ cup green onions, corn, black beans, ar tomatoes to cooked quinoa.

06. Drizzle remaining 2 tbsp lime juice and 1 tbs olive oil over quinoa. Season to taste with sa and toss to coat. Use remaining green onions a a garnish.

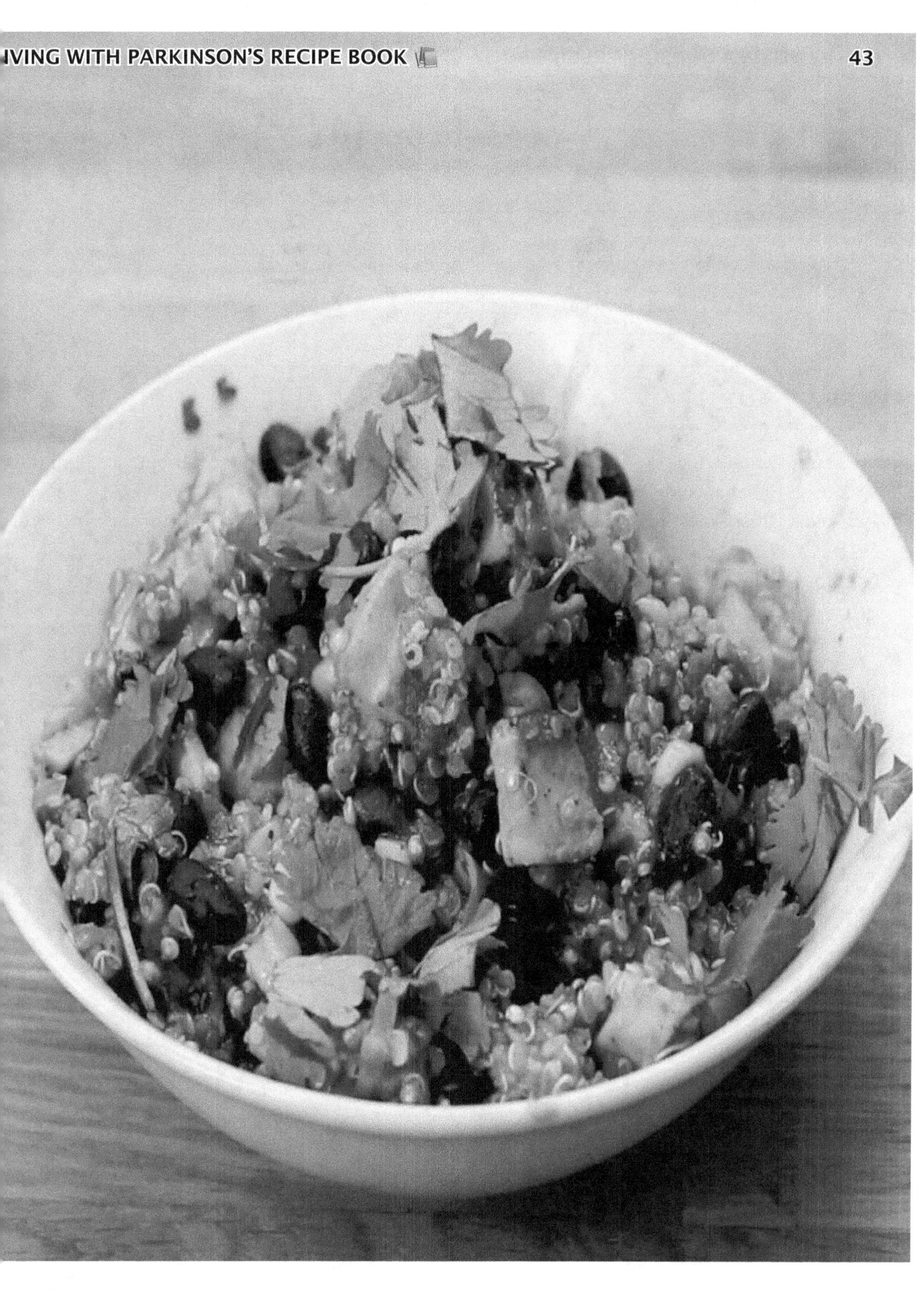

Banana Berry Smoothie

Ready In About 5 min

Servings 04

Ingredients

- 2 cups Orange juice
- 2 each Banana, cut in half
- 2 cups Blueberries, frozen
- 1 cup Strawberries, frozen
- 2 tbsp Honey

Direction

01. In a blender, purée all ingredients until smooth

02. Pour into an airtight container and keep refrigerated.

03. Enjoy!

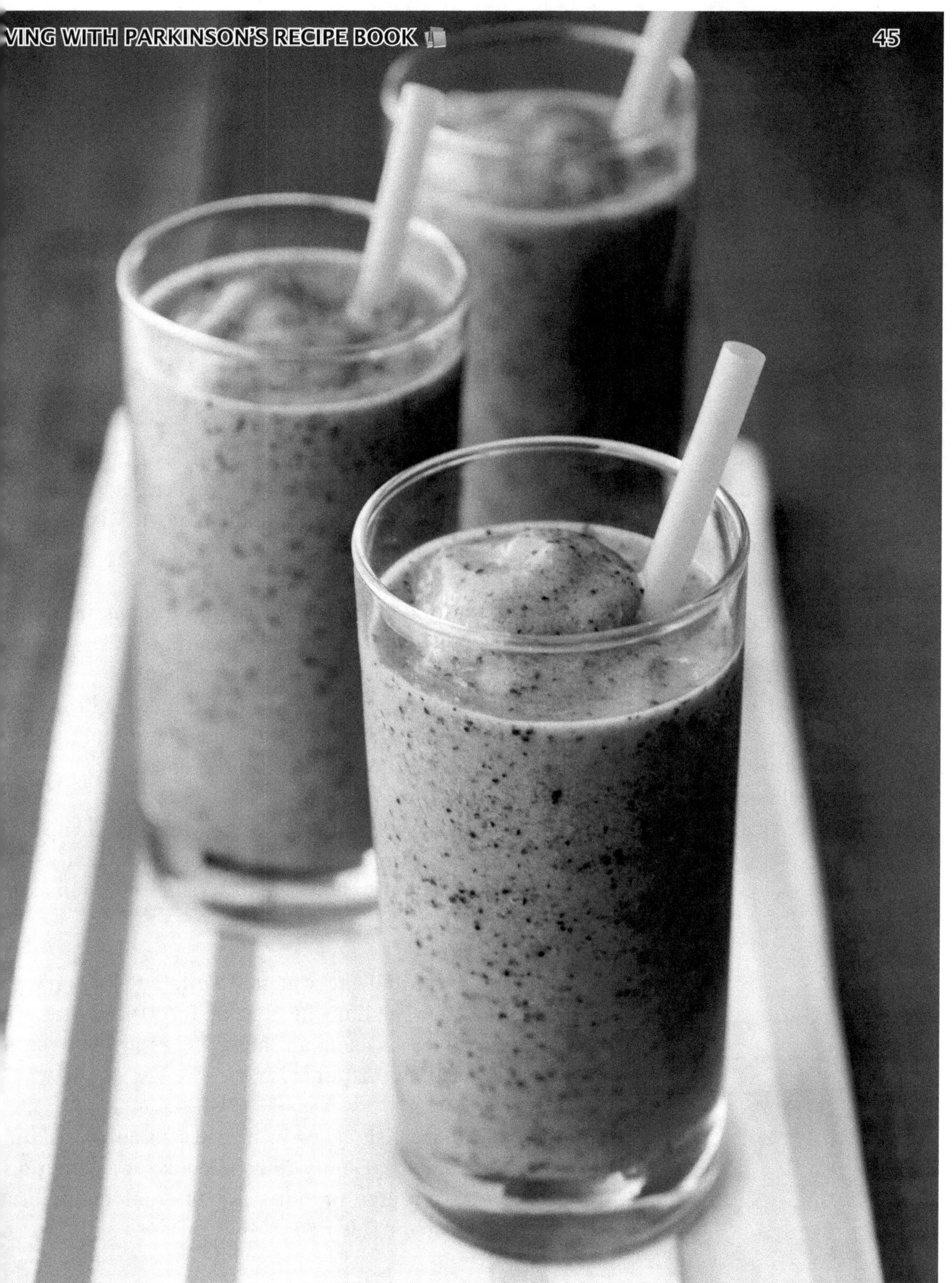

Salmon Fish Cakes

Ready In About 50 min

Servings 04

Ingredients

- 4 each Green onion, chopped
- 1 tbsp Dried dill
- ¼ tsp Salt
- ¼ tsp Black pepper
- ½ tsp Cayenne pepper (optional)
- 1 tsp Onion powder
- 1 each Lemon, zest and juice
- 1 each Egg
- 1 can Black beans, drained and rinsed
- 3 -213g cans Salmon, drained
- ½ cup All-purpose flour
- ¼ cup Vegetable oil

Direction

01. Combine green onion, dill, salt, black peppe[r] cayenne pepper, onion powder, lemon zest an[d] juice, and egg in a medium bowl. Mix until we[ll] combined.

02. Using a fork, slightly mash beans in a sma[ll] bowl and add to egg mixture.

03. Flake salmon into large pieces with a for[k]. Incorporate into bean and egg mixture. Add ¼ cup flour and stir until combined.

04. Form into 8 cakes. Approximately ½ cup (- cup of the mixture for each cake. Gently pre[ss] together to hold and dust cakes with remainin[g] flour.

05. Heat half the vegetable oil, 2 tbsp in fry pa[n] over medium heat.Bake for 10 minutes, fl[ip] potatoes using a spatula and return to oven f[or] another 15 minutes.

06. Place fish cakes in heated pan and cook for minutes. Gently flip and cook for an addition[al] 5 minutes or until the internal temperatu[re] reaches 160°F (71°C).

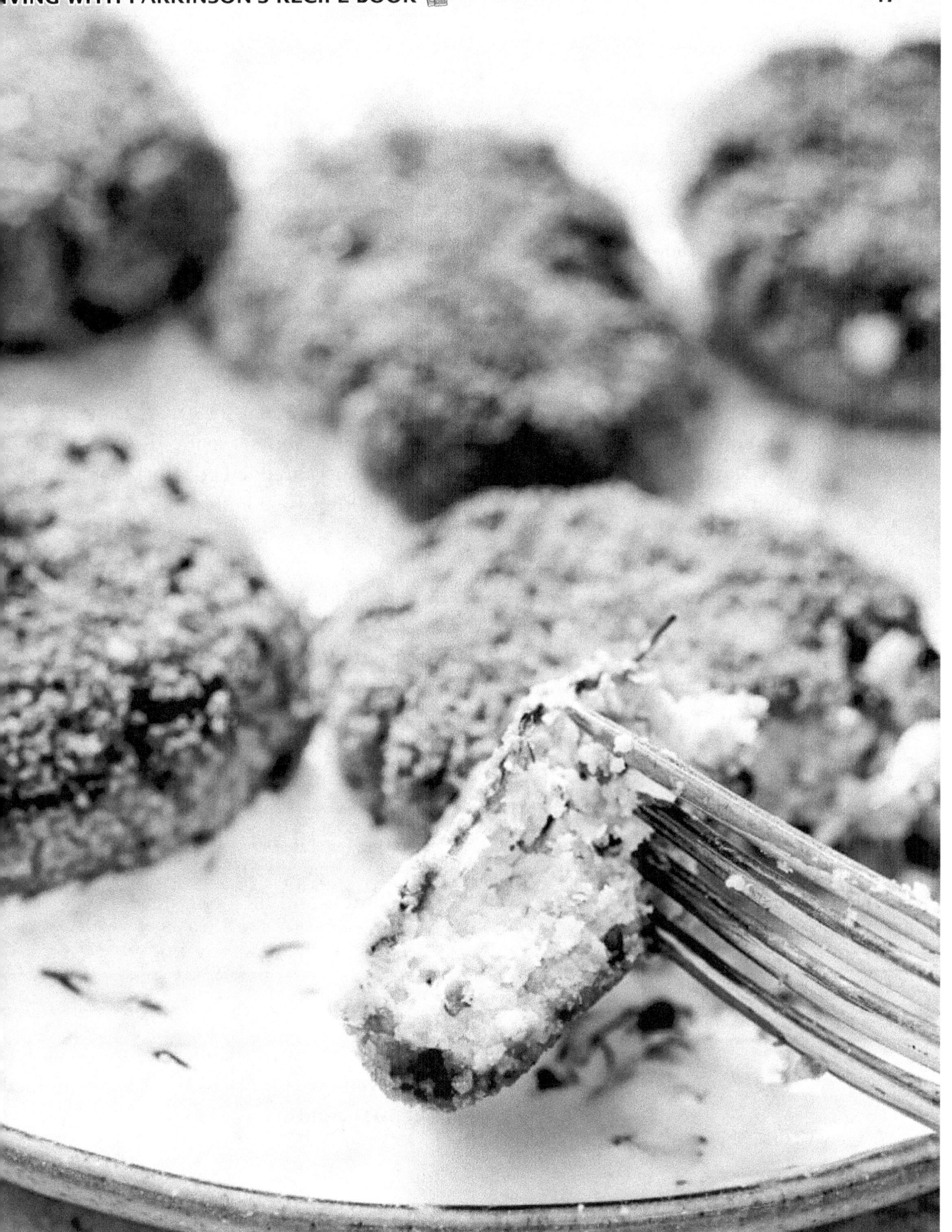

Pina Colada Cupcakes

Ready In About 35 min

Servings 12

Ingredients

Cupcakes:
- 1¼ cup All-purpose flour
- ¼ cup Dried shredded coconut, unsweetened
- ½ cup Sugar
- ½ tsp Baking powder
- ½ tsp Baking soda
- ¼ tsp Salt
- ½ cup Coconut milk
- ¾ cup Crushed pineapple, canned and well drained. Reserve juice.
- ½ cup Pineapple juice, from drained pineapple
- ¼ cup Vegetable oil
- ½ tsp Vanilla extract

Coconut Glaze:
- 1 cup Confectioner's sugar
- 1 tbsp Butter, softened
- 3 tbsp) Coconut milk
- 1 tsp Vanilla extract

Direction

01. Preheat oven to 350°F (180°C). Line cupcak pan with liners and set aside. In a large bowl combine flour, shredded coconut, sugar, baking powder, baking soda and salt.

02. In a separate bowl, whisk together coconut milk, pineapple juice, vegetable oil and vanilla extract. Add wet ingredients to dry ingredient and stir to combine.

03. Lastly, gently stir in crushed pineapple until just incorporated. Using an ice cream scoop divide batter into lined pan.

04. Bake for 25-30 minutes or until inserted toothpick comes out clean. Allow to cool in par for 5 minutes, and then transfer to a wire rack to cool completely.

Coconut Glaze

05. Whisk confectioner's sugar, butter, coconut milk and vanilla extract together until combined. About 30 seconds.

06. When cupcakes are completely cooled, fros with 2 tsp of icing each.

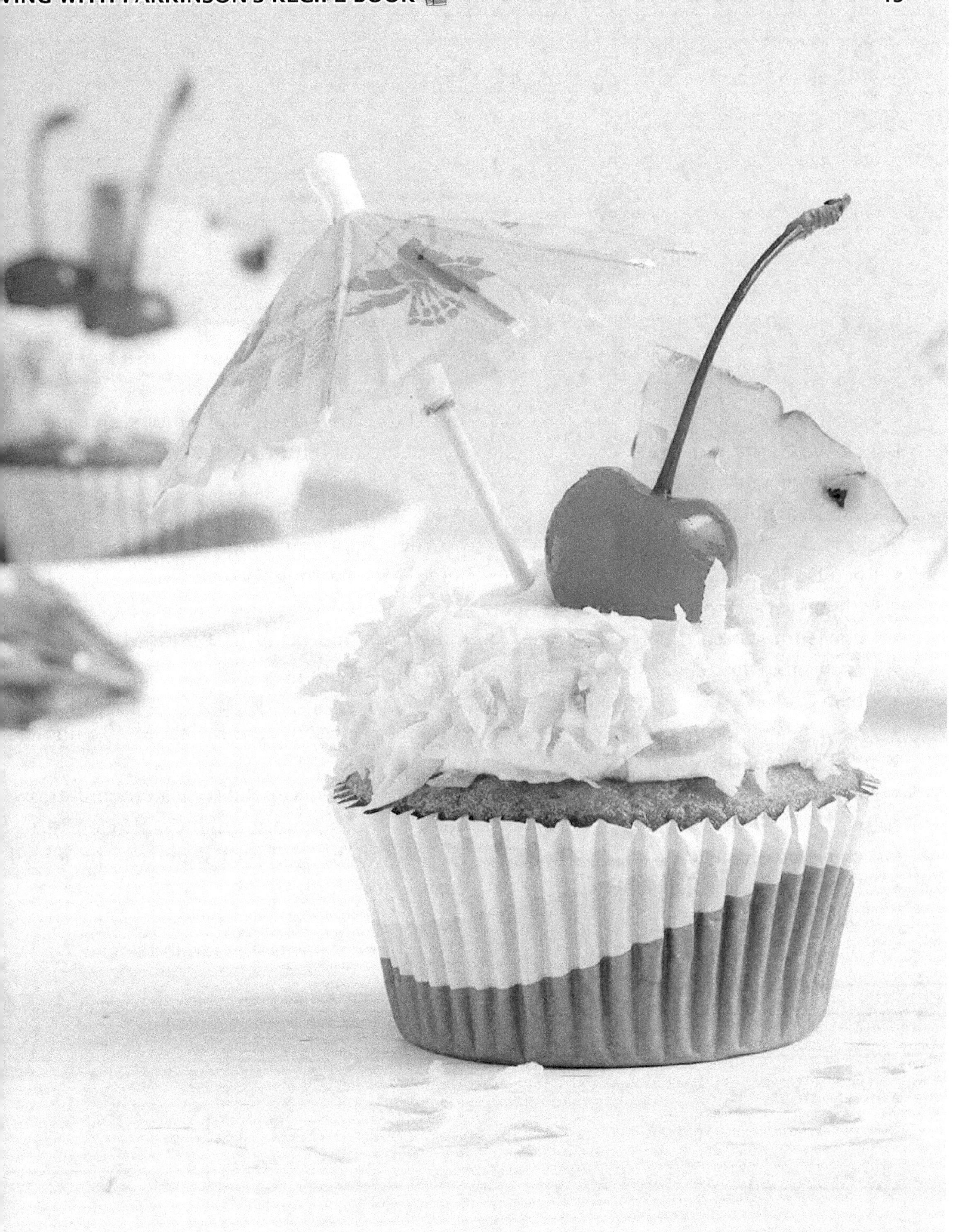

Vegetable Chili

Ready In About 35 min

Servings 04

Ingredients

- 1 each Onion, chopped
- 4 cloves Garlic, minced
- 1 tbsp Vegetable oil
- 1 can Bean medley, canned, rinsed
- 1 can Diced canned tomatoes, with juices
- 1 cup Corn, frozen
- 1 each Lime, juiced
- 2 tbsp Chili powder
- 1 each Jalapeño pepper, seeded, diced (optional)
- 2 tsp Paprika powder
- 1 tsp Salt
- 2 cups Tomato juice
- 1 ½ cups Textured vegetable protein
- 4 pieces Green onion, chopped

Direction

01. In a large pot, sauté the onions and garlic vegetable oil until translucent.

02. Add beans, tomatoes, corn, lime juice, ch powder, jalapeño, paprika, salt and toma juice. Mix thoroughly.

03. Cover pot and bring to a boil. Stir and redu heat to a simmer.

04. Simmer while covered for about 20 minutes.

05. Stir in textured vegetable protein and allow cook for 3 – 5 more minutes. Season to tast An additional ½ cup of water can be added chili is too thick.

06. Stir in green onion. Season to taste.

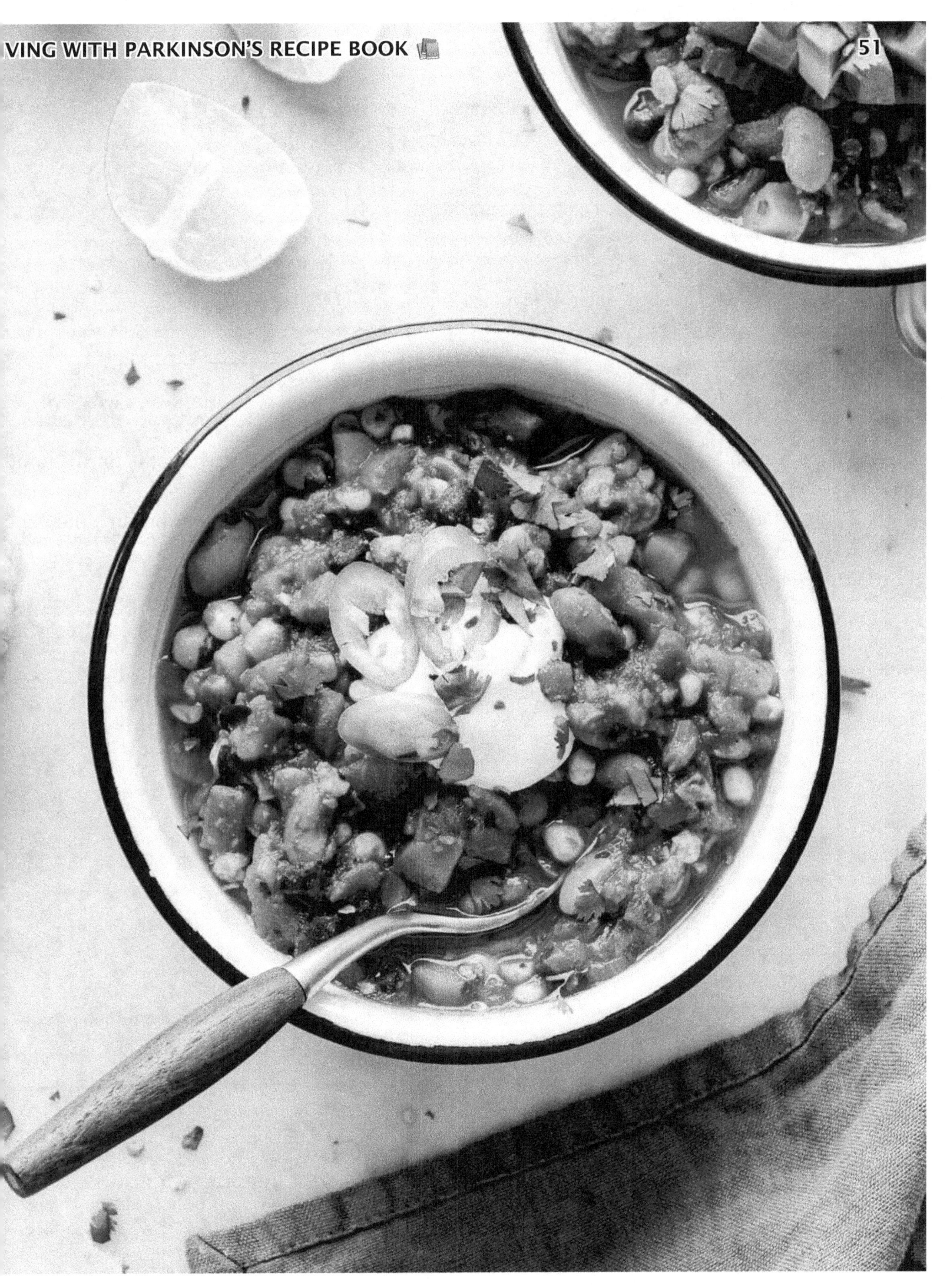

Strawberry Mango Smoothie

Ready In About 05 min

Servings 04

Ingredients

- 2 cups Almond milk
- 1 each Banana, cut in half
- 2 cups Mango, frozen
- 2 cups Strawberries, frozen
- 2 tbsp Honey

Direction

01. In a blender, purée all ingredients until smooth

02. Pour into an airtight container and kee refrigerated.

03. Enjoy!

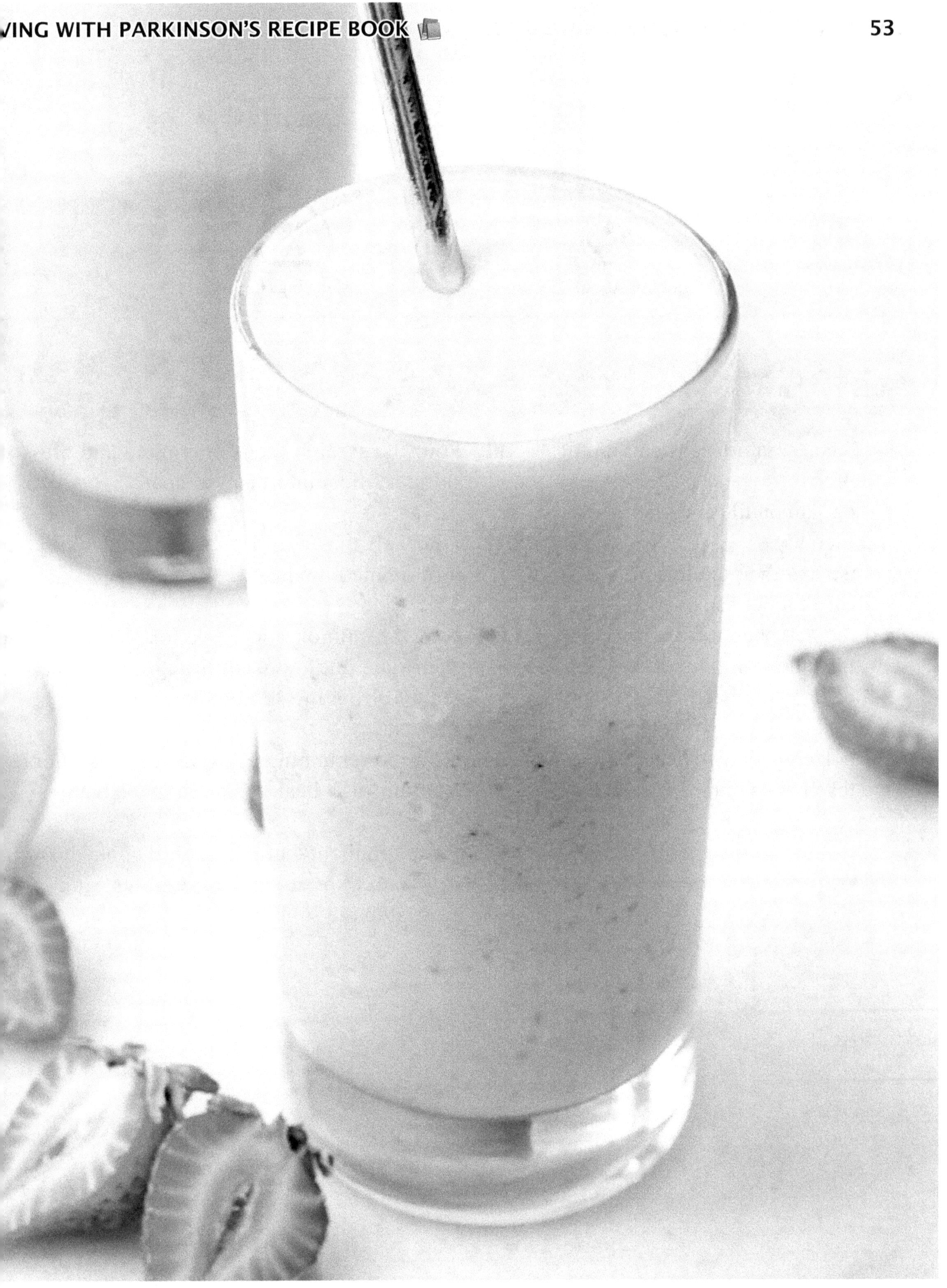

Sesame Crusted Salmon

Ready In About 25 min

Servings 02

Ingredients

- 1/8 cup sesame seeds plus a little more
- 4 oz salmon fillets wild, preferably
- 1 tsp extra virgin olive oil
- 1 carrot julienned or sliced thin
- 1 red bell pepper cored, seeded, thinly sliced or julienned
- 4 oz baby portabella mushrooms sliced
- 1 bok choy thinly sliced
- 5 tbsp low-sodium soy sauce

Direction

01. Pour the sesame seeds on a plate and press t salmon fillets into them to coat.

02. Pour half of the oil into a non-stick skillet a turn on medium heat.

03. Add the salmon and cook for 3-4 minutes each side, until cooked through. When cooke remove from the skillet and set aside.

04. Heat the remaining oil in the same skillet ov medium-high heat and add the vegetables.

05. Saute for about 4 minutes, until cooked. Drizz soy sauce over the vegetables and enjc alongside the salmon.

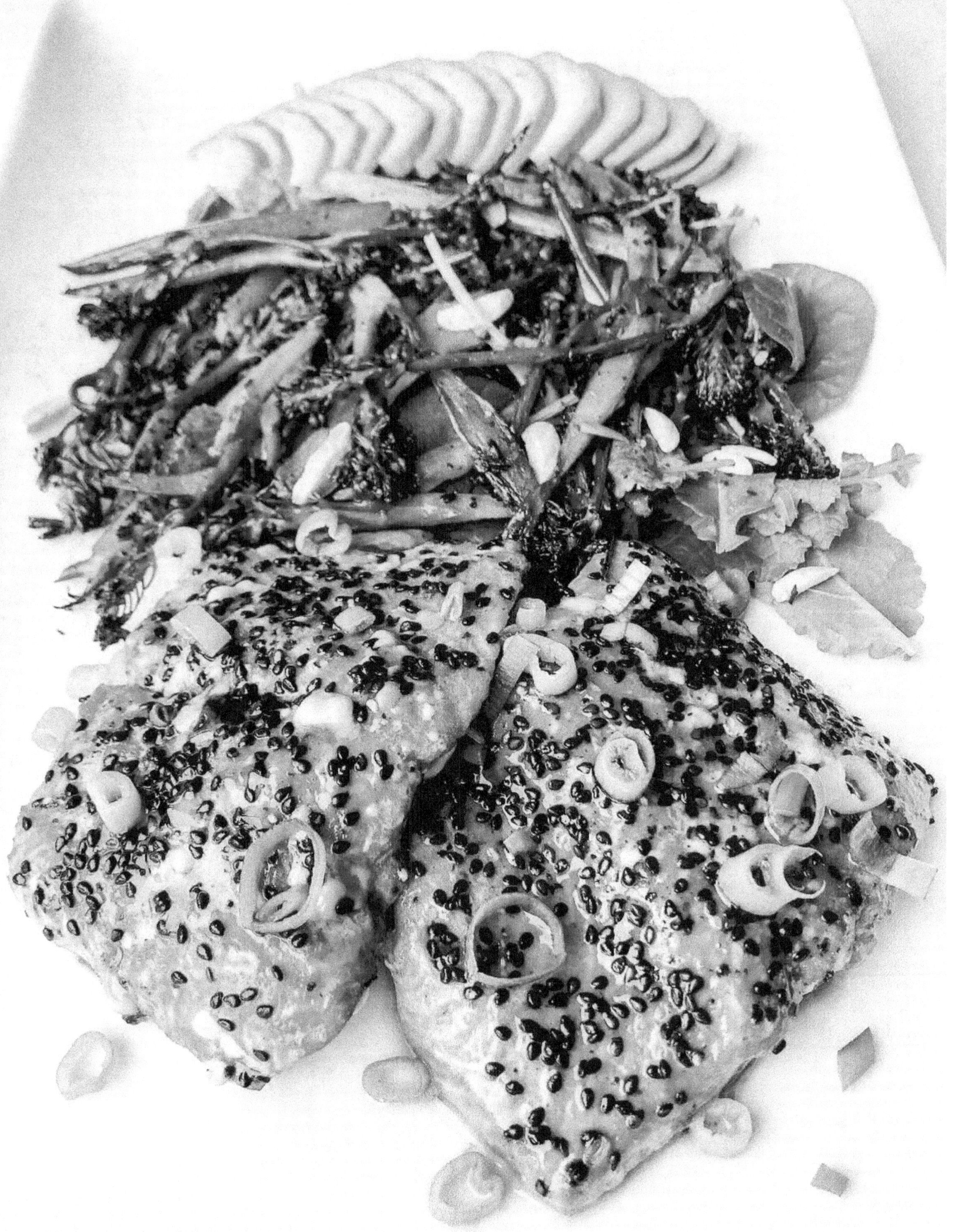

Lemon Ginger Turmeric Tea

Ready In About 05 min

Servings 02

Ingredients

- 1 ½ qt water
- ½ a lemon, sliced or rough chopped (or more to taste), rind included
- 1" ginger root, rough chopped (or more to taste)
- big dash of turmeric
- big dash cinnamon
- 2 tbsp maple syrup (more or less to taste)

Direction

01. Fill a 2 quart pot about ¾ full with water.

02. Add in all other ingredients and bring to a boil on the stove.

03. Reduce heat and simmer for 10 minutes. The remove from heat and allow the drink to cool off. Strain into a glass jar.

04. Chill overnight in the fridge for an iced tea (or enjoy hot straight away)!

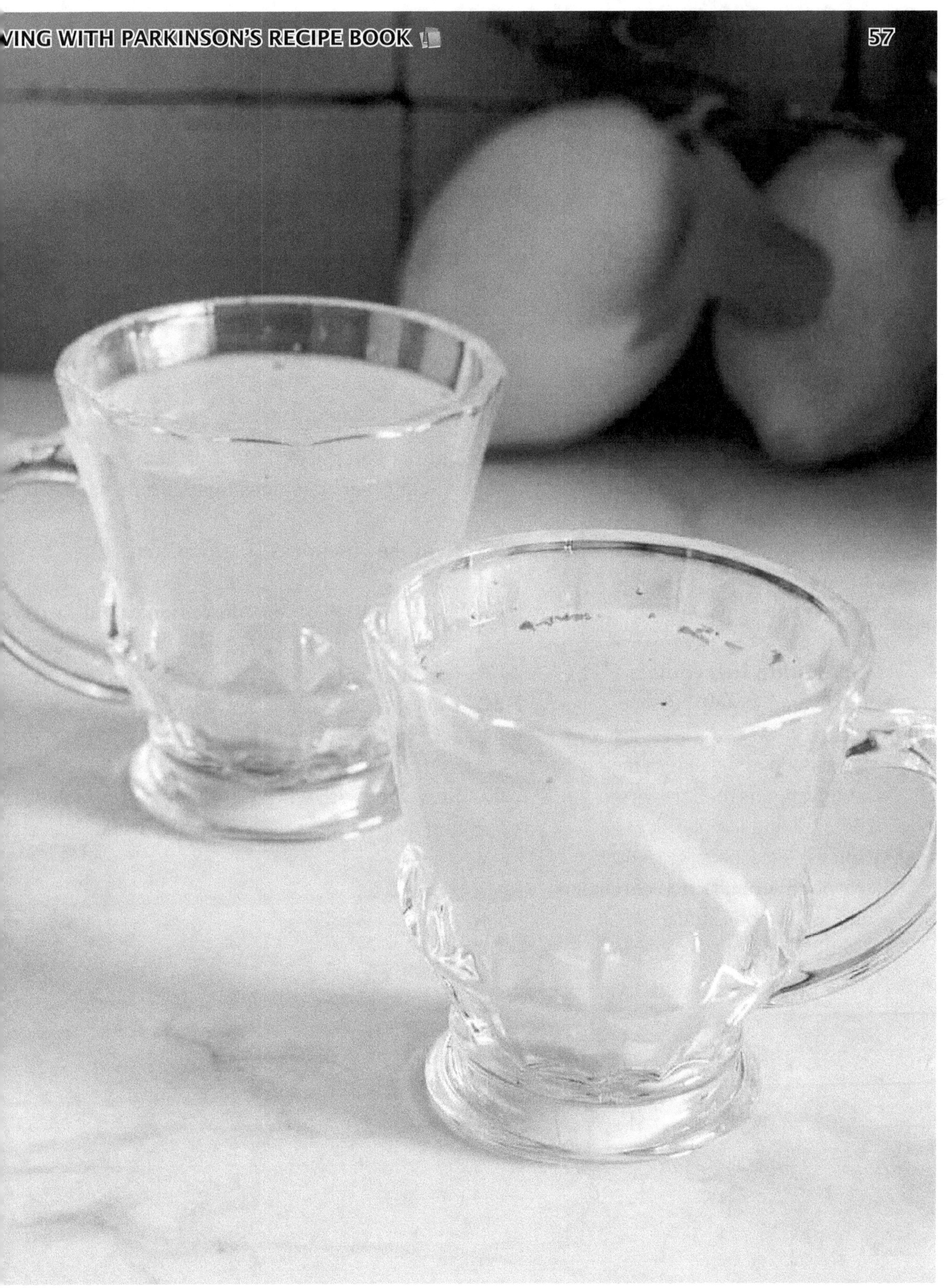

Chickpeas Breakfast Recipe

Ready In About 05 min

Servings 02

Ingredients

- 1 cup freshly boiled chickpeas.
- ½ cup carrots, cut into small squares.
- ½ cup cucumber, cut into small squares.
- Tahina and sumac for garnishing

Seasoning Ingredients
- 1 teaspoon freshly crushed garlic.
- 1 teaspoon apple cider vinegar.
- 5 tablespoons of extra-virgin olive oil and lemon juice.
- **Spices** ½ teaspoon sea salt, ½ teaspoon ground dried coriander and ½ teaspoon sumac.
- 1 tablespoon ground cumin.

Direction

01. Put the chickpeas, olive oil, lemon, apple cid vinegar, garlic, spices, and cumin, then stir.

02. Heat the chickpeas if they were cold.

03. Add the rest of the ingredients and stir we until they are mixed.

04. Garnish the plate with tahini, sumac, ar parsley, as desired.

05. Serve hot with whole-grain bread, labneh sauc and a hot cup of your favorite drink.

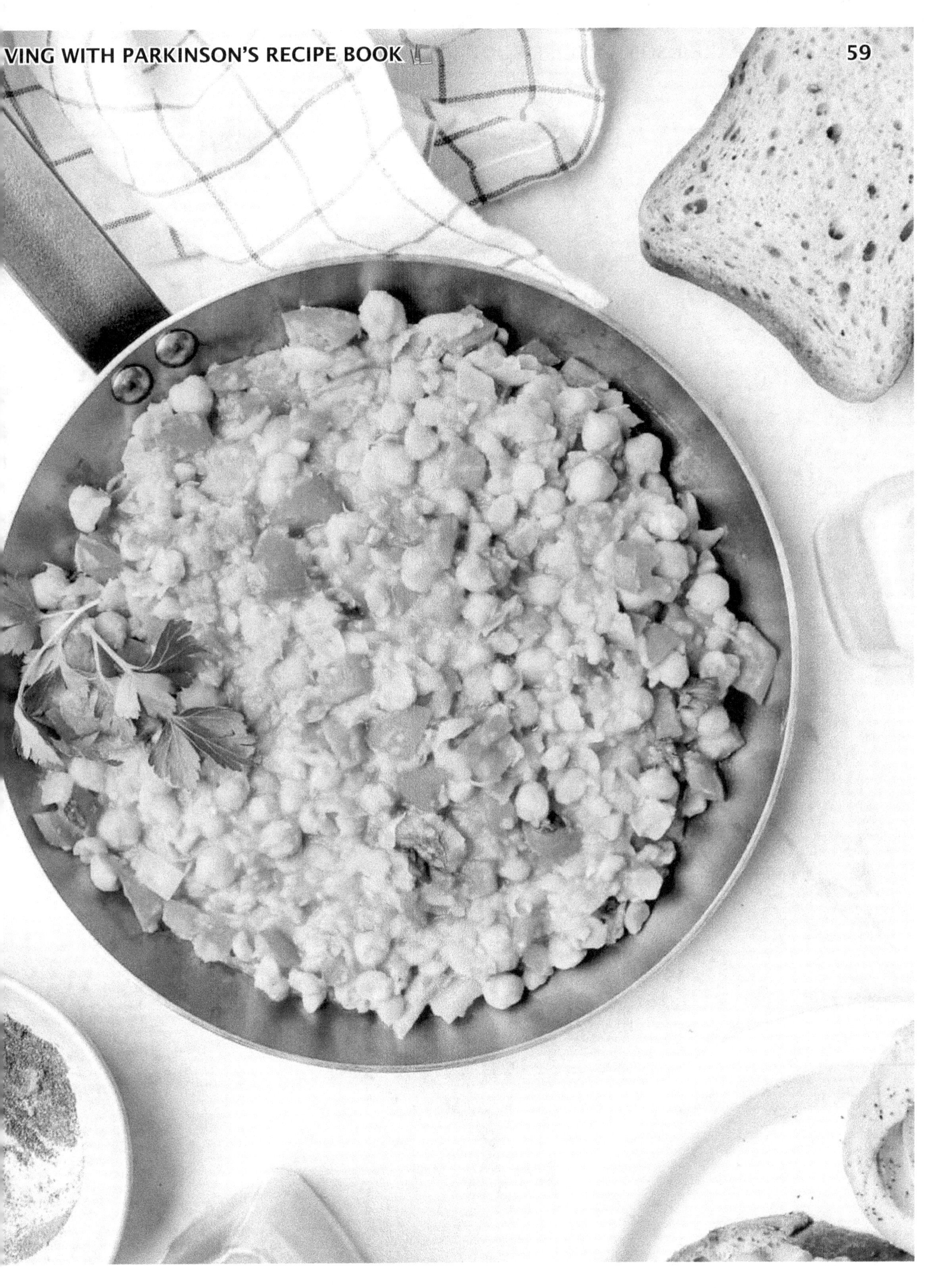

Overnight Oatmeal Recipe

Ready In About 10 min

Servings 02

Ingredients

- 1/2 cup rolled oats or quick-cooking oats
- 1 cup plant milk (almond, cashew, etc.)
- 1/2 cup of blueberries
- 1 tablespoon chia seeds
- 1 tablespoon agave nectar, maple syrup or honey
- 1 small handful of slivered almonds
- Cinnamon (to taste)

Direction

01. In a small Mason jar, mix all ingredient together except for a few blueberries.

02. Place the remaining blueberries on top of th mixture.

03. Let stand in refrigerator for 1 hour or overnight

04. Enjoy!

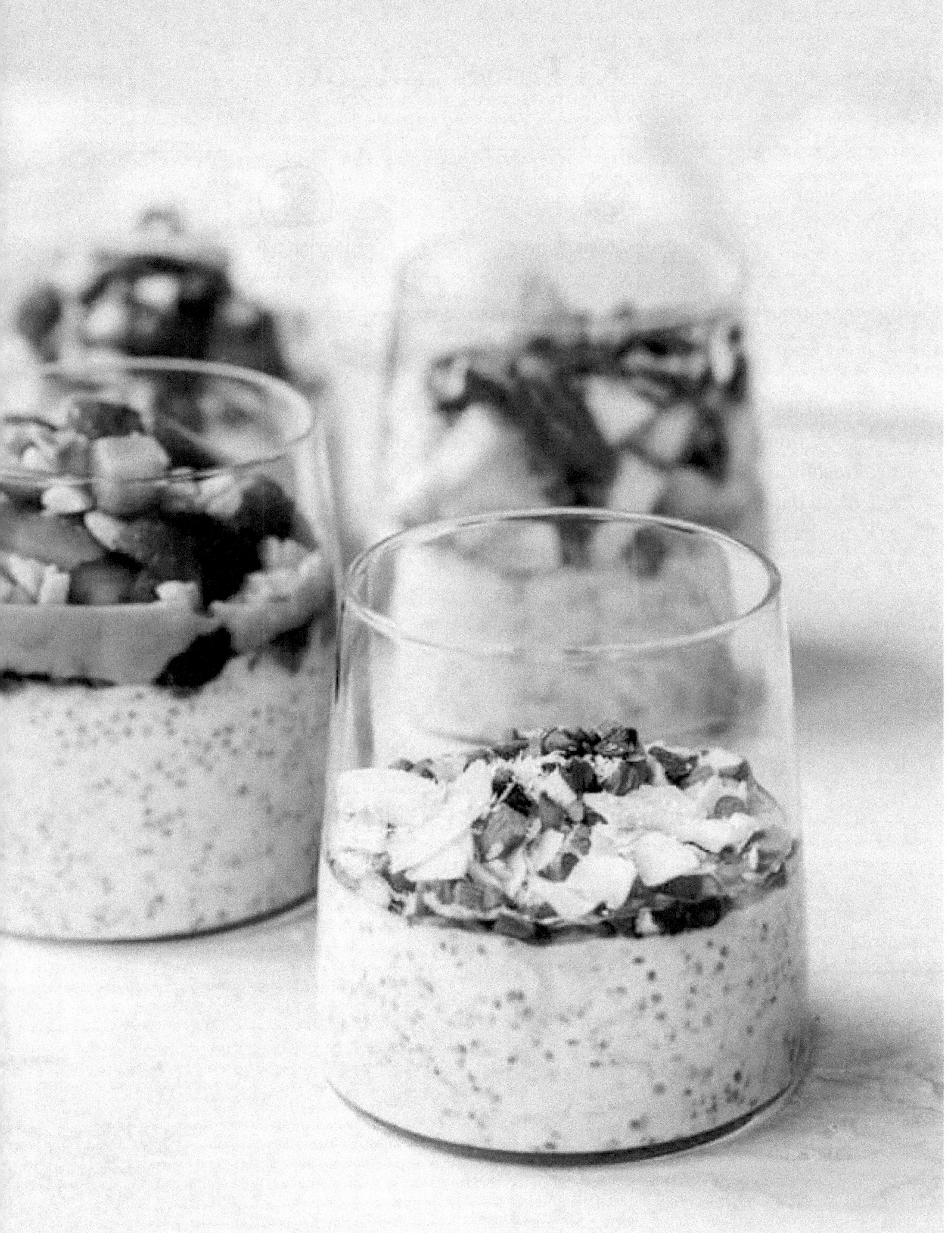

Sea Moss Smoothie

Ready In About 05 min

Servings 02

Ingredients

- 1/4 cup Sea Moss Gel
- 2 cups almond milk
- 2 fresh or dried figs
- 2 dried dates
- 1 ripe banana

Direction

01. Place sea moss gel in a high-speed blender wi almond milk, figs, dates, and banana.

02. Process until smooth and creamy, enjoy

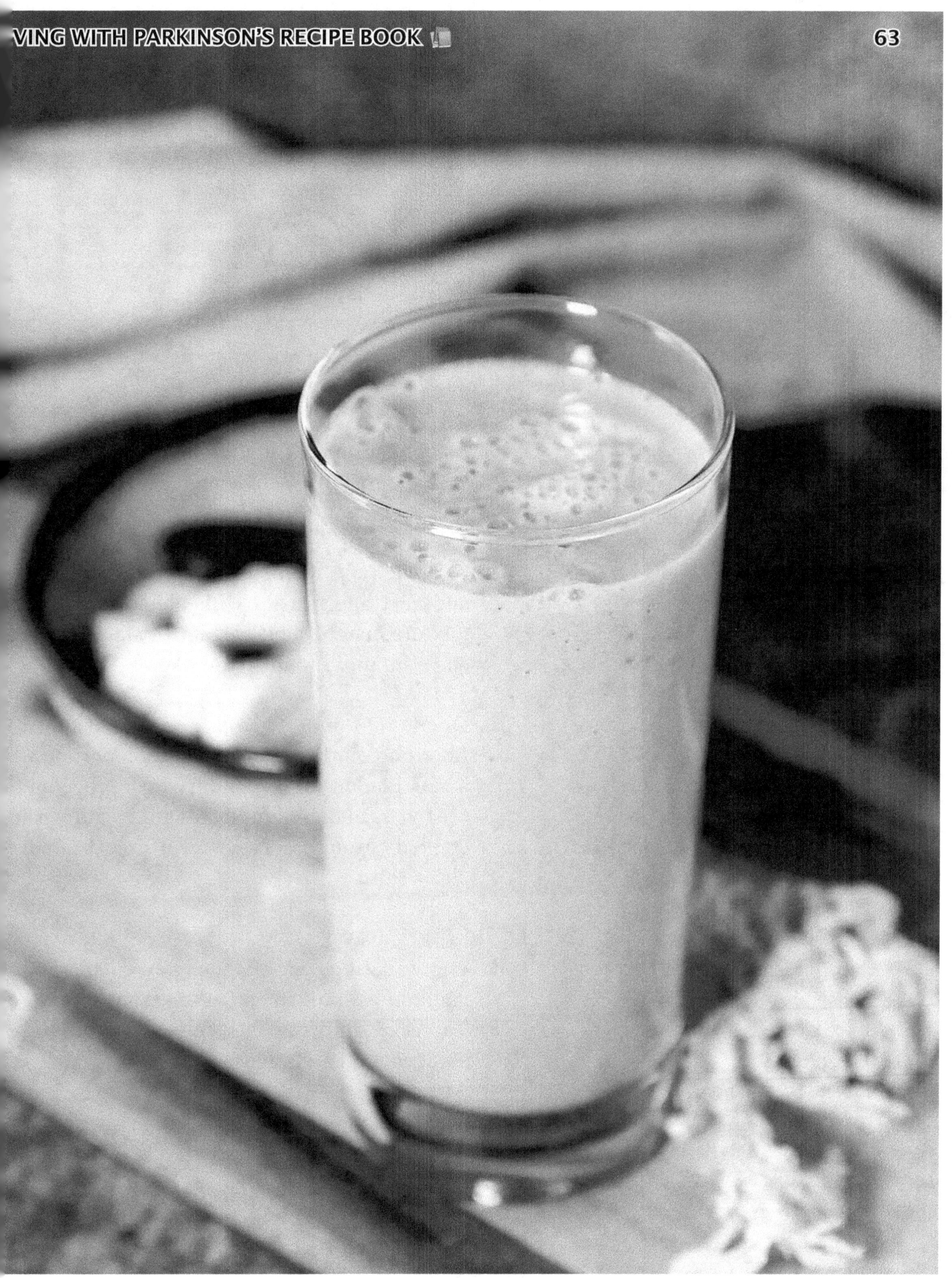

Thai fishcakes with zingy salsa

Ready In About 60 min

Servings 02

Ingredients

- 150-200g white fish
- 4 spring onions, chopped
- 1 inch fresh root ginger, grated
- 1 tsp Thai green curry paste
- 1 egg, beaten
- 2 tbsp chopped coriander
- 1 tbsp flour
- Juice and zest of a lime
- Black pepper
- 1 tsp coconut oil

For the salsa
- ½ cucumber, finely chopped
- ½ red onion, finely chopped
- 2 medium tomatoes, chopped
- 1 red pepper, finely chopped
- ½ fresh chilli, finely chopped
- 2 tbsp fresh coriander, chopped
- 1 tbsp chives, chopped
- Juice of 1 lime
- 1 tbsp olive oil
- Freshly ground black pepper

Direction

01. Finely chop the fish and place in a large bow with the spring onions, ginger, curry paste, fis sauce, egg and coriander.

02. Mix well and then stir in the flour, lime juic and zest and season with black pepper. Th mixture may be a bit wet at this stage. You ca add a bit more flour if you like.

03. Divide into four generous portions. Put a littl flour on your hands and form each portion int a ball. Flatten slightly and fry in the coconut o for five to eight minutes until golden brown an cooked through.Serve with a green salad o zingy salsa.

For the salsa

04. For the salsa, place all the ingredients in a bow and mix well together. Season to taste.

05. To serve, pile the salsa high on your plate alongside the fishcakes.

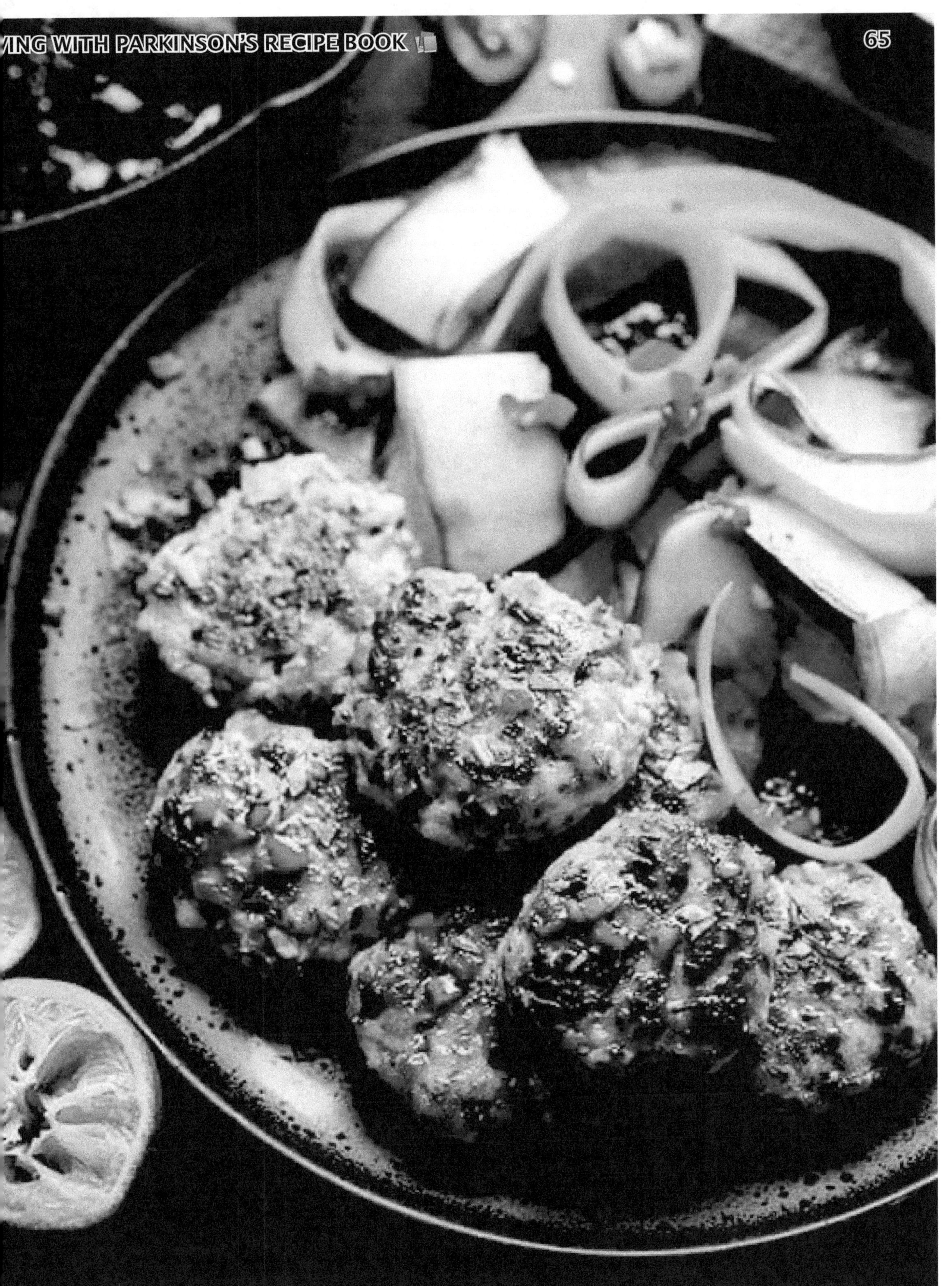

Cinnamon nectarines with vanilla scented yoghurt

Ready In About 30 min

Servings 02

Ingredients

- 1-2 tsp agave syrup
- 2 nectarines, halved with stone removed
- ½-1 tsp ground cinnamon
- ½ vanilla pod
- 2 tbsp Greek yoghurt

Direction

01. Preheat your oven to 180C/350F/Gas 4.

02. Drizzle a little agave syrup over each nectarine half and sprinkle with cinnamon.

03. Cover with tinfoil and bake for 15-20 minutes until soft.

04. Slice the vanilla pod lengthways and, with the tip of a sharp knife, scrape out the seeds and stir into the Greek yoghurt.

05. Serve the nectarines hot or cold with a drizzle of agave syrup and a dollop of the vanilla scented Greek yoghurt.

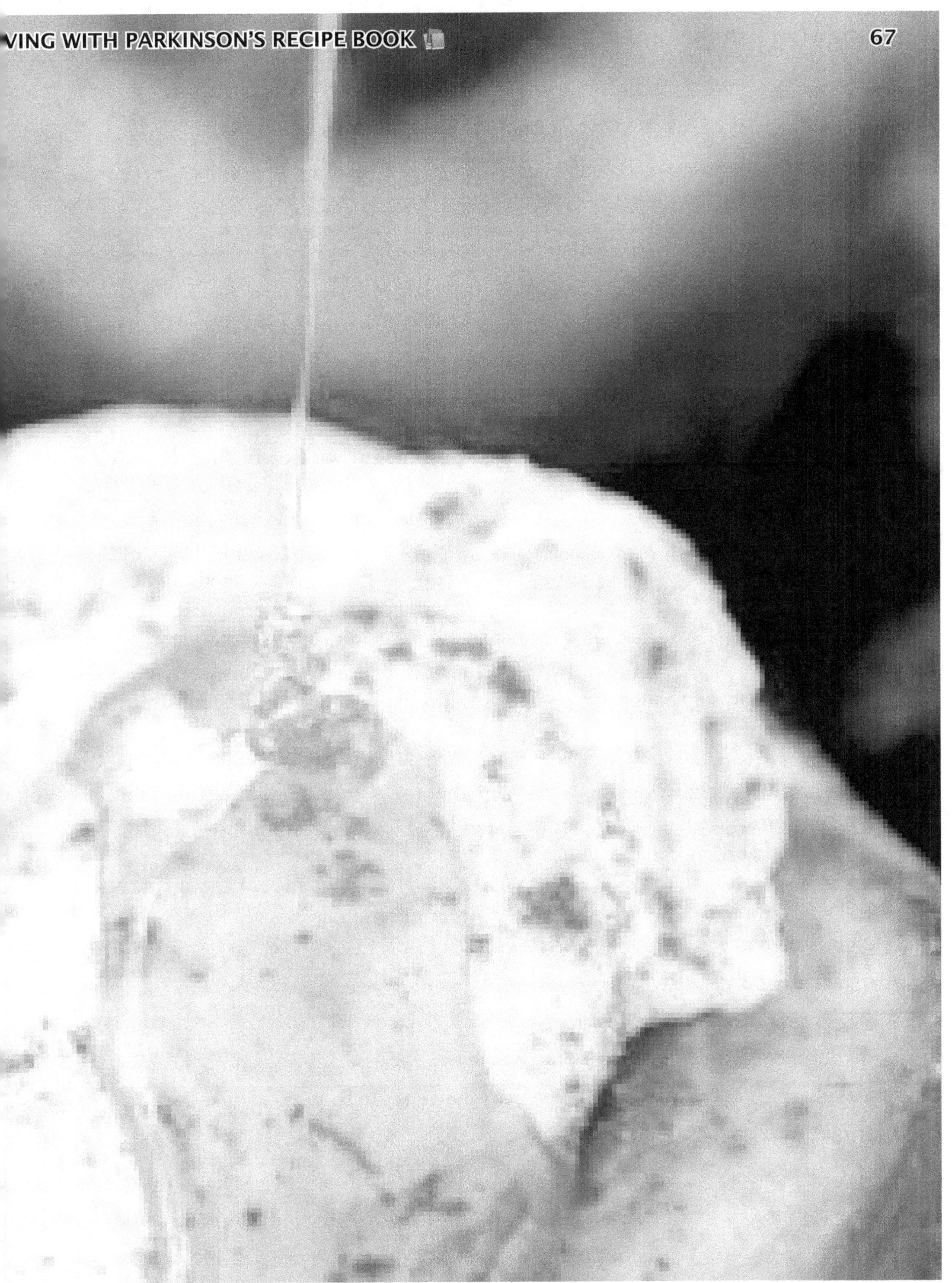

Mediterranean chicken tagine

Ready In About 60 min

Servings 04

Ingredients

- 500g chicken breast
- 100ml vegetable stock
- 1 aubergine
- 1 courgette
- 1 yellow pepper
- 1 red pepper
- 150g mushrooms
- 1 red onion
- 1 tablespoon freshly chopped garlic
- 1 rosemary twig
- 200g precooked chickpeas
- 300g tomato purée
- 1 tablespoon of 'ras el hanout' spice mix
- 1 halved lemon
- 200g brown rice
- Extra virgin olive oil

Direction

01. Boil the brown rice in slightly salted water.

02. Fry the chicken in the tagine with extra virgi olive oil, together with the onion and freshl chopped garlic over a medium heat (a pan wit cover is a simple alternative if you don't have ceramic tagine).

03. Add the vegetable cubes and stir

04. Soften with the vegetable stock before addin the tomato purée, and then the precooke chickpeas.

05. Season with the ras el hanout spices and add th lemon segments.

06. Cover the tagine and allow to simmer on gentle heat for 20 minutes .

07. Uncover after 20 minutes, remove the lemo and season to taste with salt.

08. Stir and serve immediately.

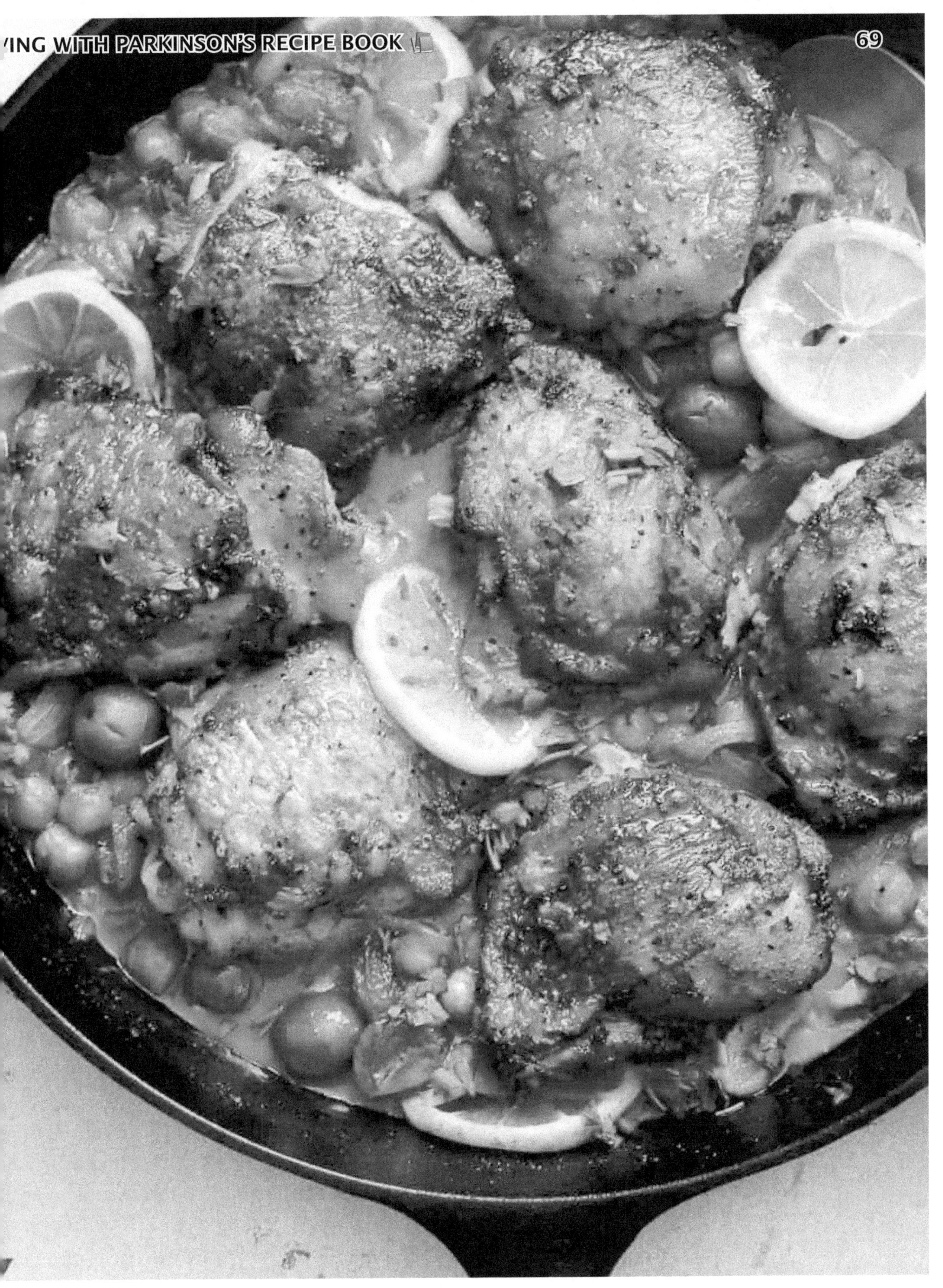

Beet Wellington

Ready In About 50 min

Servings 04

Ingredients

- 140g fresh, organic beetroots
- 100g mushrooms
- 4 sheets 20x20cm puff pastry
- 3 tbsp breadcrumbs
- 2 shallots (roughly chopped)
- 2 pinches of aniseed
- 1 clove of garlic (roughly chopped)
- 1 tbsp of cut sage
- 1 tbsp tomato purée
- 1 aubergine (diced)
- 1 egg yolk (mixed with 1 tbsp oil and water)
- 1 tsp poppy seeds (optional)
- Sunflower oil
- Flour
- Pepper
- Salt (optional)

Direction

01. Preheat oven to 180°C. Place the beetroots in an oven dish and brush them with sunflow oil. Roast the beetroots in the oven for minutes. Remove the skin from the beetroot Mix sunflower oil with pepper, 1 pinch aniseed and sage. Brush the oil mixture on the beetroots. Sprinkle some salt on to (optional). Heat sunflower oil in a frying pa and fry the aubergine, shallots, garlic an mushrooms. Add the tomato purée and a splas of water, stir thoroughly. Add the breadcrumb sage and 1 pinch of aniseed. Cook on a low he for ten minutes, stirring from time to time.

02. Purée the mixture in a blender, leave to coo Pre-heat the oven to 220°C. Place sheets pastry on a cool, floured surface. Brush th edges of the pastry with the mixture of eg yolk, water and oil. Place ½ tbsp of breadcrumb in the middle of each sheet. Spread the puré mixture over the sheets of pastry. Place th beetroot on top of the purée mixture. As tightl as possible, fold the pastry sheets over the puré and beetroot. Turn the pastry over and brush eg yolk over the top. Sprinkle poppy seeds over th dough (optional). Bake the Beet Wellington f 20 minutes, until golden brown.

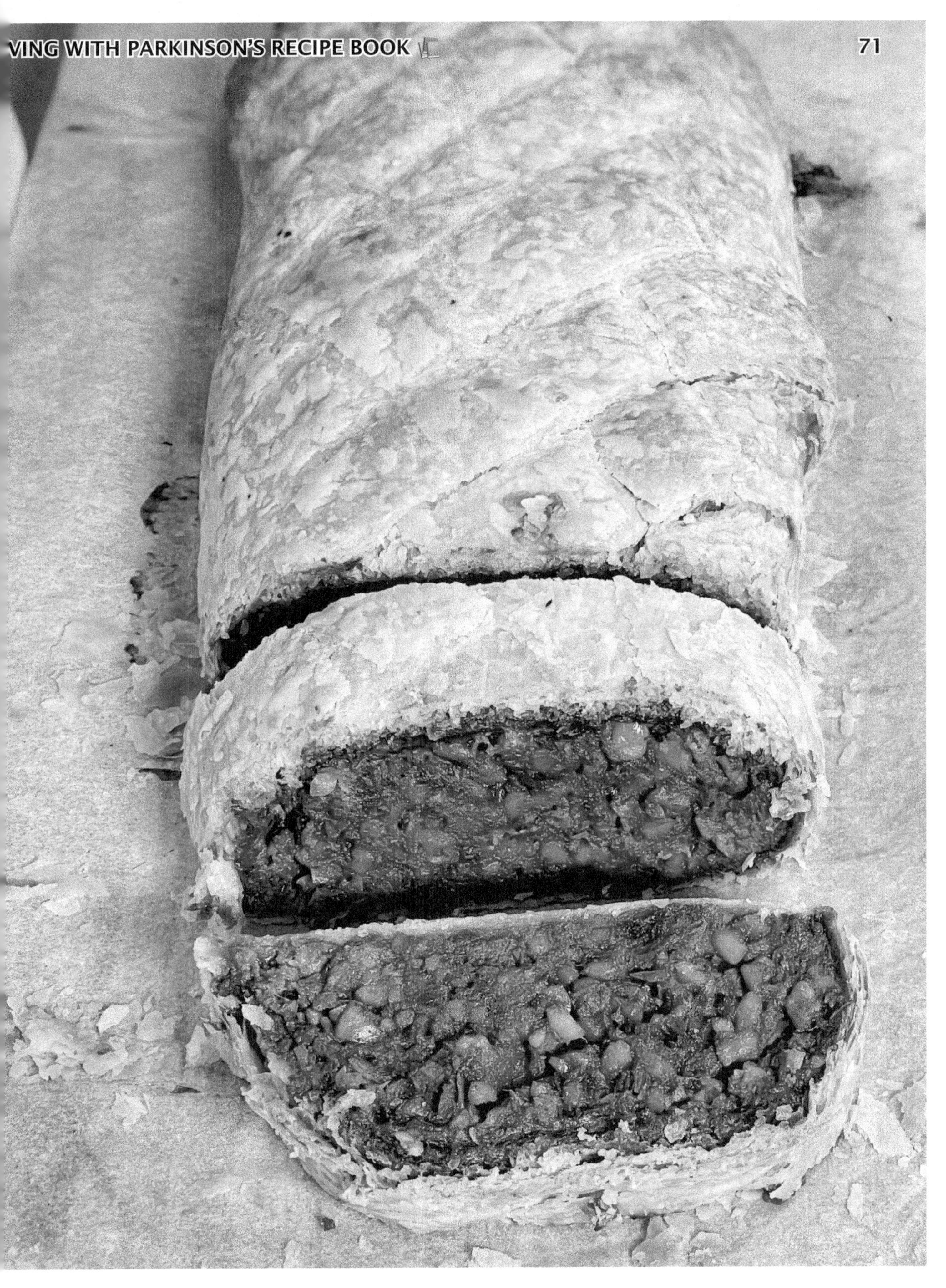

Chicory Apple Juice

Ready In About 05 min

Servings 02

Ingredients

- 2 cups papaya, diced and seeded
- 1 apple, with no seeds
- 2 cups fresh chicory
- 150 ml cold water

Direction

01. Add all the ingredients in the electric mixer i order.

02. After that, mix at high speed for 30-60 second until there is a smooth juice.

03. Enjoy!

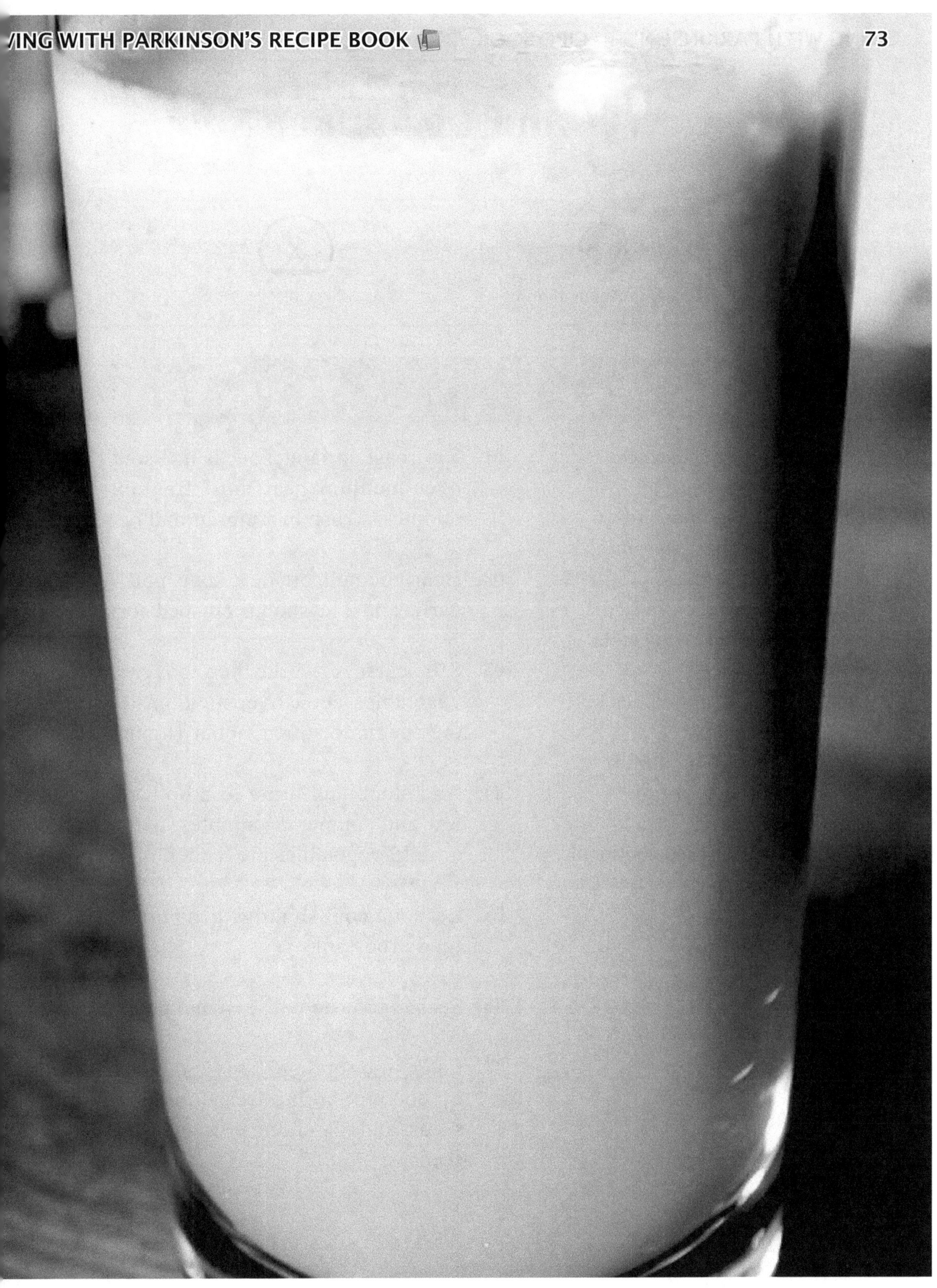

/ING WITH PARKINSON'S RECIPE BOOK

Carrot and Coriander Soup

Ready In About 45 min

Servings 04

Ingredients

- 1 tablespoon coriander seeds
- 1 tablespoon coconut oil
- 2 pounds carrots about 14-16 whole carrots, peeled, trimmed and cut into 1" pieces
- 1 small clove garlic crushed
- 6 cups low sodium vegetable stock
- salt and freshly ground black pepper to taste
- 3 tablespoons coconut milk
- fresh cilantro for garnish, optional
- toasted pumpkin seeds optional

Direction

01. Dry roast coriander seeds in a small frying pa over medium heat until fragrant, about 1 minutes. Crush in a mortar and pestle.

02. Heat coconut oil in a soup pot. Add carrot garlic and 2 teaspoons crushed coriander seed

03. Stir carrots well, then cover pot and l vegetables cook over medium-low heat unt they begin to soften, about 10 minutes.

04. Add stock and bring to a boil; reduce heat low and simmer 20 minutes, partially covere or until vegetables are tender.

05. Let soup cool slightly, then puree in blender food processor.

06. Season to taste with salt and pepper.

07. Ladle into serving bowls and garnish with swi of coconut milk, fresh coriander, pumpki seeds, and remaining crushed toasted coriande seeds.

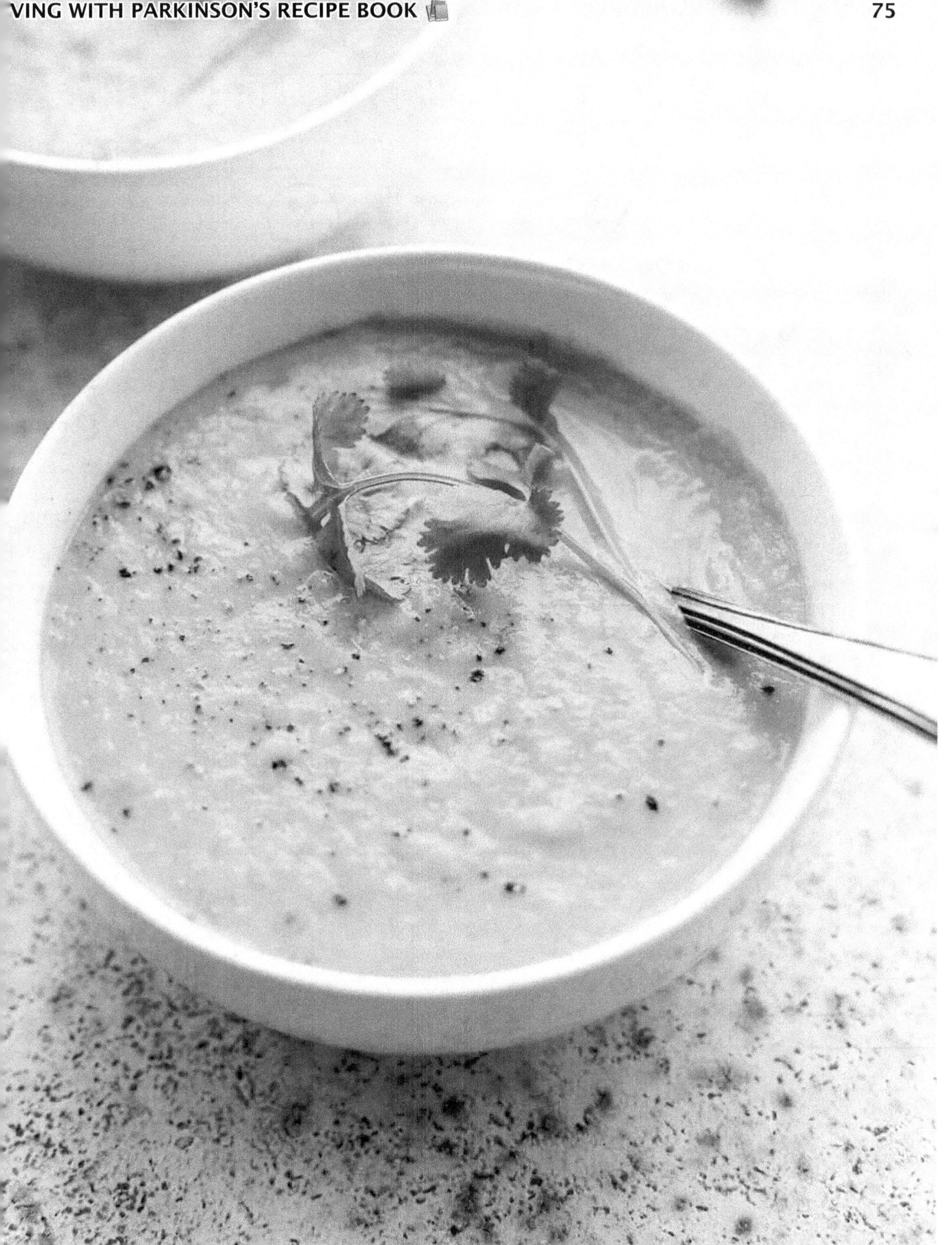

Miso Soup with Carrots and Tofu

Ready In About 20 min

Servings 02

Ingredients

- 2 cups water
- 1/10 tsp salt , or to taste
- 1/3 medium carrot, cut into 1/4-inch dice
- 1/8 cup shiro miso (white fermented soybean paste)
- 1/6 cup 1/4-inch dice of silken tofu (3 oz)

Direction

01. Bring 5 1/2 cups water with salt to a boil in 2-quart saucepan.

02. Add carrot, then reduce heat and simmer covered, until tender, about 3 minutes. Remov from heat.

03. Whisk together shiro miso and remaining 1/ cup water in a small bowl until smooth, the whisk into carrot mixture. Add tofu and serv immediately.

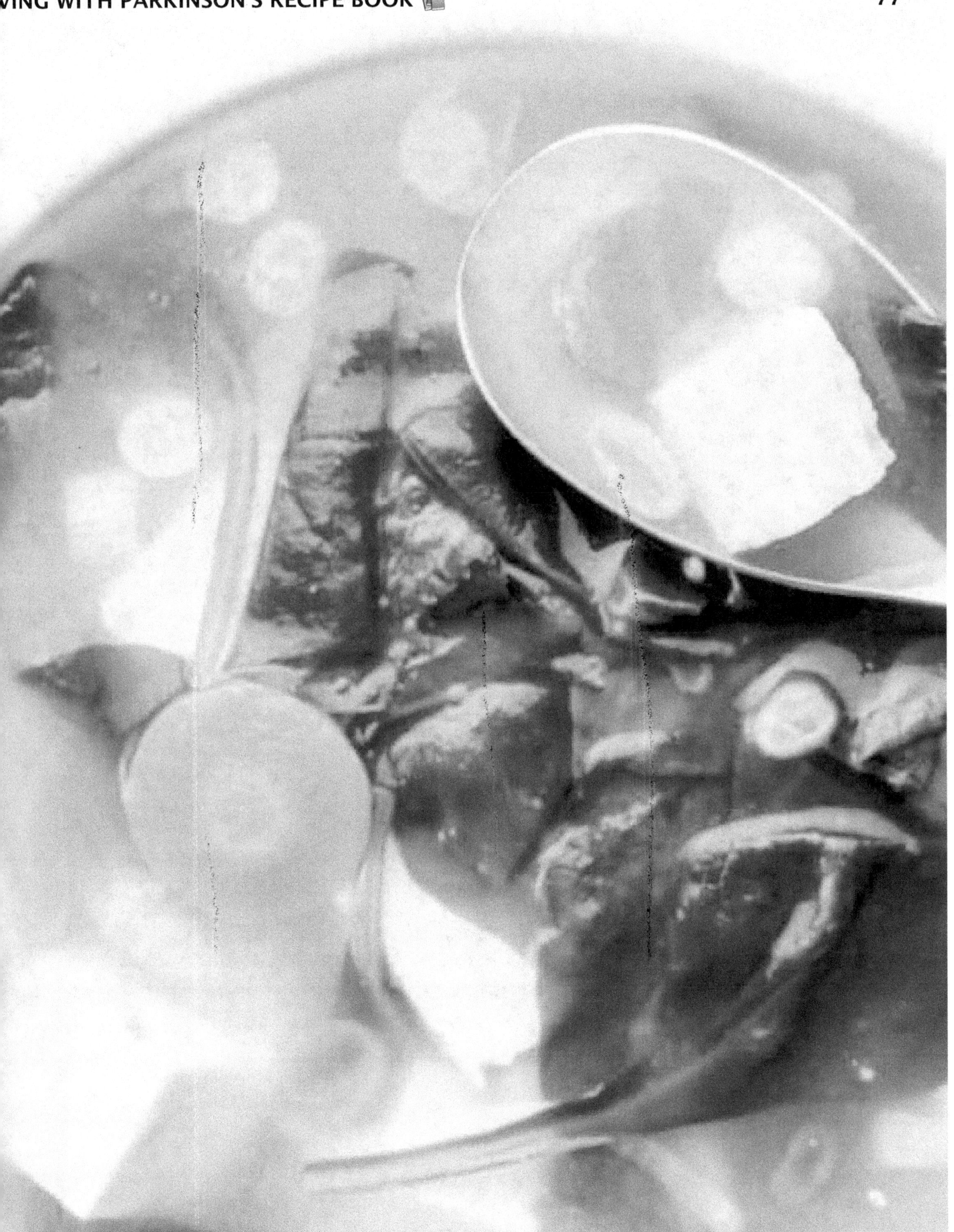

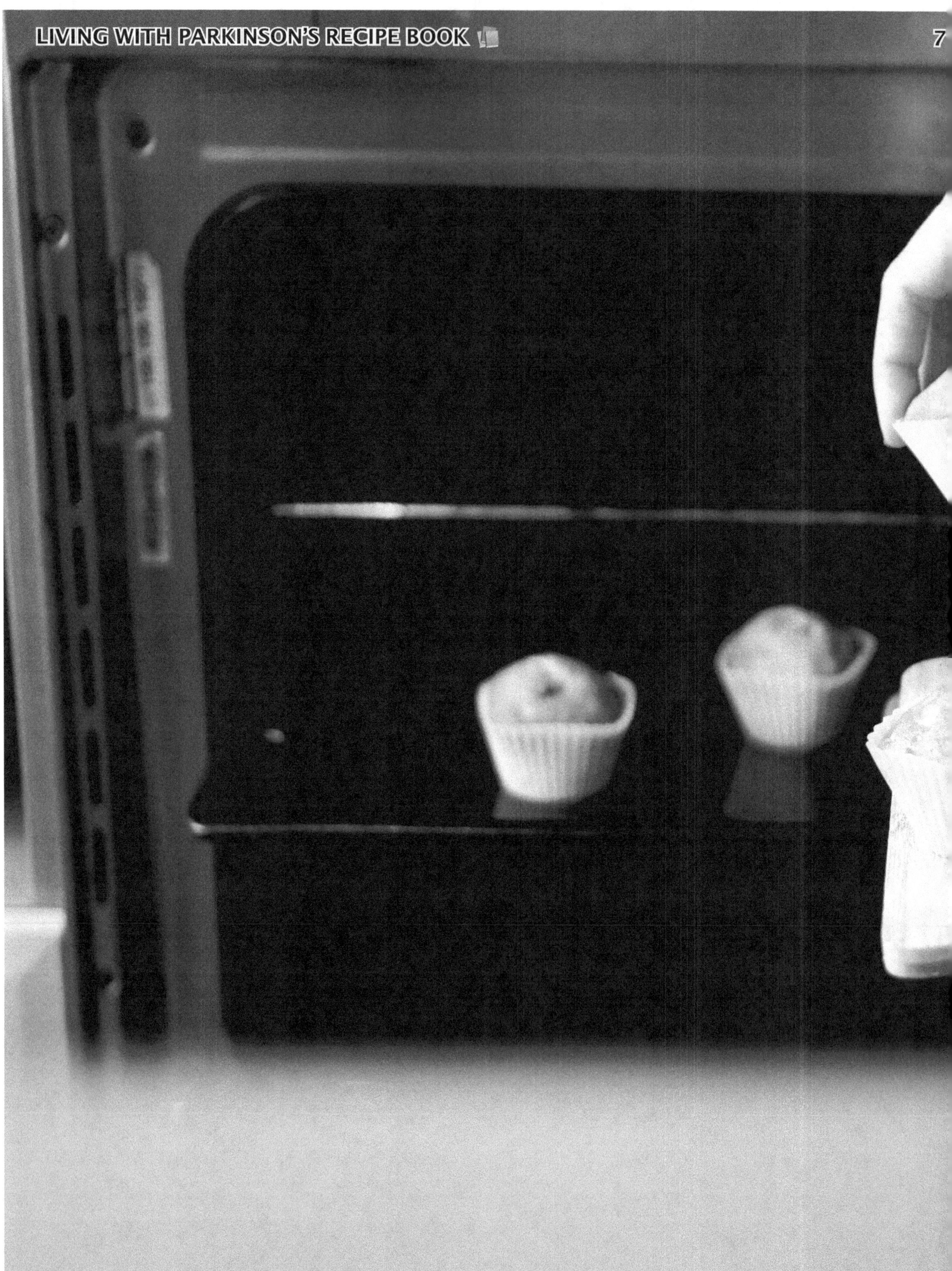

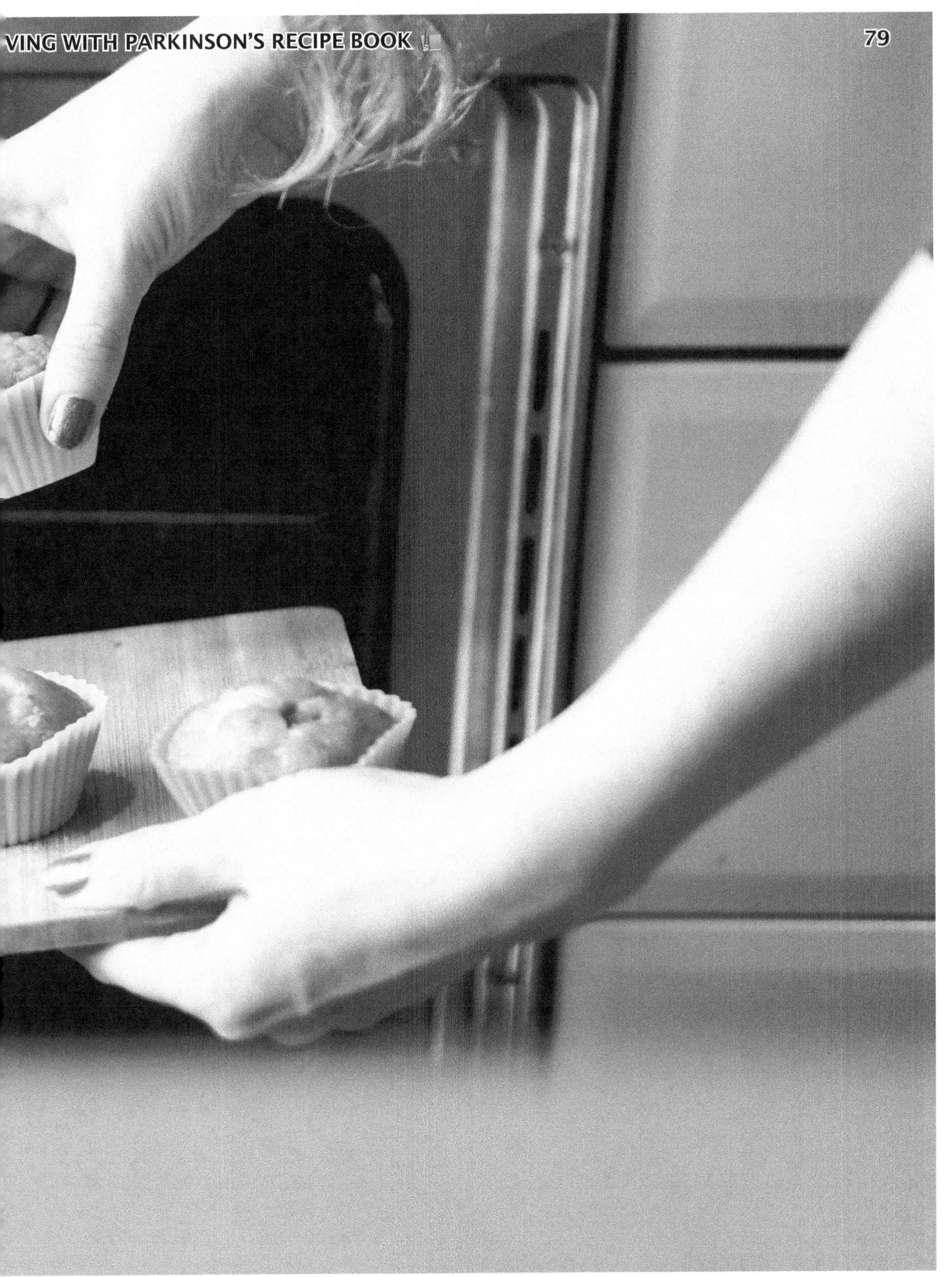